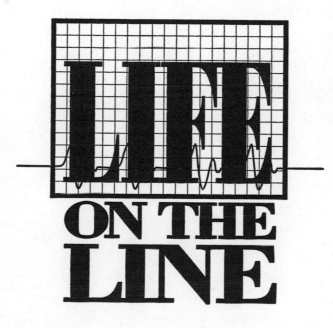

*Critical Choices **You** Must Face*

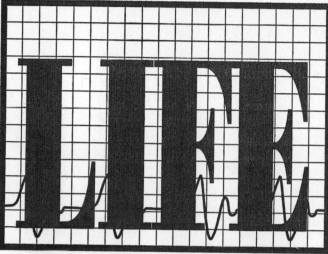

LIFE
ON THE
LINE

ELIZABETH R.
SKOGLUND

World Wide Publications
A ministry of the Billy Graham Evangelistic Association
1303 Hennepin Ave., Minneapolis, MN 55403

Life on the Line

© 1989 Elizabeth R. Skoglund

World Wide Publications is the publishing ministry of the Billy Graham Evangelistic Association.

Unless otherwise indicated, Scripture quotations are taken from the Authorized King James Version of the Bible.

Scripture quotations marked NIV are taken from The Holy Bible, New International Version. Copyright © 1973, 1978, 1984 International Bible Society. Used by permission of Zondervan Bible Publishers.

Scripture quotations marked RSV are taken by permission from the Revised Standard Version Bible, © 1946, 1952, 1971, 1973 National Council of Churches of Christ in the U.S.A., New York, New York.

Scripture quotations marked Moffatt are taken from *The New Testament, A New Translation*, by James Moffatt, Harper and Brothers, New York, 1935. Courtesy of Harper and Row Publishers.

Scripture quotations marked Weymouth are taken from *Weymouth's New Testament in Modern Speech*, by Richard Francis Weymouth, as revised by J. A. Robertson. Published by special arrangement with James Clarke and Company Ltd., London. Reprinted by permission of Harper and Row Publishers, Inc. and James Clarke and Company Ltd.

Scripture quotations marked TLB or *The Living Bible* are taken from *The Living Bible*, © 1971 Tyndale House Publishers. Used by permission.

Library of Congress Catalog Card Number: 89-050951

ISBN: 0-89066-178-2

Printed in the United States of America

Contents

(Where mention is made of people involved in professional counseling situations, names, gender, and nonessential details have been altered to protect their privacy.)

For my father, Ragnar Emanuel Skoglund.

For the unknown little girl at Belzec who went to her death in the concentration camp saying: "It's so dark and I was being so good."

For the Swedish diplomat Raoul Wallenberg, who showed that even in the middle of such disillusionment, one life can make a difference.

For Swedish ambassador Per Anger, who has helped keep this message alive.

For those everywhere who in the common light of everyday life resist evil and make a decision to love—and thereby make a difference.

The doctor, . . . if not living in a moral situation . . . where limits are very clear . . . is very dangerous.

—*Auschwitz Survivor*

Those who do not remember the past are condemned to relive it.

—*Santayana*

The veils of the future are lifted one by one, and mortals must act from day to day.

—*Sir Winston Churchill*

Acknowledgments

Many years ago, Robert Wilson of Keswick, the "dear old man," as missionary Amy Carmichael was fond of calling him, said to her as they rode in a gig along a Cumberland road,

"Thee must never say . . . thee must never even let thyself think, 'I have won that soul for Christ.'"

And he pulled up the old horse, Charlie, and stopped near a stone-breaker who, squatting beside his pile of stones, was hammering steadily.

"I will tell thee a story," the dear old man said, pointing with his whip to the stone-breaker who tapped stolidly on and never looked up. "There was one who asked a stone-breaker at work by the roadside, 'Friend, which blow broke the stone?' And the stone-breaker answered, 'The first one, and the last one, and every one between.'"[1]

Charles Spurgeon told of a "French farmer whose crops were so large that he was accused of magic. The man immediately brought forth his stalwart sons and said, 'Here is my magic.'"[2]

No work for God is accomplished in isolation. As a writer I am used to the idea that writing is a solitary task. But as I began work on this book I realized that it was different than any other writing I have undertaken. Much of the material has been far from pleasant to confront, and there has been a sense of the reality of spiritual warfare. Although not wanting to appear over-dramatic, I sent out a request for prayer along with a return slip for those who desired to commit themselves to pray.

The response was overwhelming; and many friends went further, sending notes, clippings, books, and tapes relating to the subject matter. Most of all, I was intensely aware of the prayer support which prevailed throughout the writing and production of this book. Sometimes I would send a prayer request to one or two people, and many of their associates would respond along with them. This was particularly true of the people at World Wide Publications and the Billy Graham Evangelistic Association; Sister Agnes Vollmann and the Cenacle in Warrensville, Illinois; University Bible Church in Westwood Village, California; East Coast Bible Fellowship in El Cajon, California; and the singles group to which I spoke several times at La Canada Presbyterian Church in La Canada, California. Dorothy Jones, a life-long friend and prayer warrior, summed up my feelings about all this prayer support when she said she had been praying "combatingly," referring to J. N. Darby's translation of Colossians 4:12: "Always combating earnestly for you in prayers. . . ."

A core group of people have been especially generous with their support. The idea of a book discussing bioethics in the context of Christian love came into being during a luncheon with Richard Baltzell. Later, because of the far-sightedness of Stephen Griffith of World Wide Publications, the project was put "into shoe leather."

Steve has continued to be an encouragement and a creative force during the writing of the book, and Bill Deckard has been faithful in editing, suggesting changes and helping to make the book into something better. I have appreciated the unique spiritual quality as well as the dedicated interest of the staff at World Wide. Cynthia Livingston and Juanita Palmer have been of personal encouragement and have provided that vital link between the author and the public.

Dr. Matthew Conolly, professor of medicine and pharmacology at the University of California at Los Angeles School of Medicine, gave helpful research direction at the outset, while Dr. Peter Roger Breggin, who is in private practice and is director of the Center for the Study of Psychiatry, in Bethesda, Maryland, gave similar assistance at the end. Rayne Wagner has been a valued research assistant, tracking down small bits of information in obscure places.

Two couples, John and Lynn Whorrall and Ken and Carolyn Connolly, have been uniquely helpful. John has faithfully read chapters and offered creative input as well as joining with his wife in consistent prayer. Ken has been tireless in locating rare pieces of biblical exposition and discussing fine points of theology. To Carolyn has fallen the task of xeroxing and mailing such information, as well as contributing insights shaped by her experience as a nurse.

Kenneth Asp, an independent researcher, provided helpful background material on the influence of psychiatry in the Third Reich. Rabbi Yitzchok Adlerstein, director of Jewish Studies at Yeshiva University in Los Angeles, made an important contribution to my thinking in the area of the sanctity of life. Dr. Ian Jones, head of obstetrics and gynecology at Scripps Clinic, La Jolla, California, contributed to technical details on alternate reproductive techniques, and added input on medical philosophy.

The Swedish consulate in San Francisco, the Netherlands consulates in New York and Los Angeles, the Austrian consulate in Los Angeles, and the Nederlandse Vereniging Voor Vrijwillige Euthanasie (Dutch Society for Voluntary Euthanasia) were generous in their help.

I am particularly indebted to certain libraries, not only for the use of books and journals, but for the helpfulness which accompanied that use: the Library of the Goethe Institute, Los Angeles; the Library of the Jewish Federation of Greater Los Angeles; the library of the Simon Wiesenthal Center for Holocaust Studies; the Burbank Public Library; Rose Memorial Library, Biola University; the Louise Darling Biomedical

Library at the University of California at Los Angeles, and Ann Newhoff, assistant librarian at the Health Science Library at St. Joseph's Medical Center in Burbank, California. My particular gratitude goes to Carole Perl, serials assistant at the Simon Wiesenthal Library, and to Aaron Breitbart, senior researcher at the Simon Wiesenthal Center.

Others, too many to list but never to be forgotten, walked the dog, brought lunch, called, wrote notes, and advised. In whatever good this book may accomplish, they will certainly share. And while some of those acknowledged may not agree with the philosophy and conclusions of *Life on the Line*, even their disagreements have been a catalyst for making it a better book.

Winston Churchill said:

> Writing a long and substantial book is like having a friend and companion at your side, to whom you can always turn for comfort and amusement, and whose society becomes more attractive as a new and widening field of interest is lighted to the mind.[3]

While this book is not long by Churchillian standards, and the topic has at times been far from comforting, writing it has been of immense personal satisfaction. I am grateful, indeed, to those who have made it possible.

Preface

I was a small child during World War II. My memories are those of a child. I remember Pearl Harbor—December 7, 1941—not so much because of its strategic importance, but because the next morning my mother told us that she had quietly slipped out of bed and prayed all night. I had not known her to do that before, so it made a deep impression on me.

Like other American children at that time, I remember choices made at the breakfast table regarding how to use the week's ration of sugar. I remember peeking through blacked-out windows, running home from the market with my mother and sister to the sound of air-raid sirens, and visiting Japanese friends in an internment camp where the guards were kind to us as we played. I remember recipes for one-egg cakes, war bonds which we bought at school, and stacks of newspapers, along with coffee cans full of bacon fat and other grease, which were collected for the war effort. I remember that certain commodities like Fleers Double Bubble Gum were not available in my town during the war. And at the end, I remember walking up and down the streets with my family and friends, banging pans in a rare expression of unbounded joy that the war was over at last.

But for me it was actually far from over. During the war

our parents had taken us to the weekly newsreel in Hollywood. The films provided heavy material for young children, and when the war ended the memories remained, seared into my brain: mass graves, mass shootings, cadaverlike bodies that were still alive, and seemingly endless stretches of film where victims were bulldozed into open graves.

Sometimes during the newsreels I closed my eyes, or my mother would gently cover them and let me know when I could look again. But I saw most of it. And I knew that somehow because these people were Jewish, this had happened to them. What I had seen in earlier newsreels of battlefields and bombings was terrifying; but what I saw of the treatment of the Jewish people, toward the end of the war when the story of the Holocaust began to break, was devastating to my childhood innocence.

The memories were revived at times during the ensuing years, like when I became friends with a concentration camp survivor, or as I discovered a book about some hero of that period like Raoul Wallenberg. When I started my private practice as a family counselor, men like Dr. Viktor Frankl, himself a death camp survivor, influenced me deeply; and again I remembered what I had seen. Then when I lost what remained of my family in a personal tragedy, it was a letter from Dr. Joseph Fabry, also a survivor of Hitler's ravages, which touched me deeply and challenged me to go on. The Holocaust may have happened when I was under seven years of age, and it may have happened "over there," but still it continued to influence my life.

As I have gone on and taught school and counseled and written books, certain social trends in America have increasingly commanded my attention: ethics based on what I *feel* rather than what I believe; the viewpoint that human life is worth only what it can produce materially; the attitude that God must conform to what I want from him if I am to believe in him. The actions which result from such thinking alarm me even more: abortion without even the acknowledgment that a human life is being destroyed; euthanasia, which at best claims to be voluntary and humanitarian and at worst becomes a way to kill those considered unworthy of life; and the health care policies of a rich yet cost-conscious society which is dangerously close to evaluating human life in terms of dollars and cents, productivity, intelligence level, and perhaps even in terms of age and race.

Then I have remembered once again those stacks of bodies in the newsreels I saw as a child. But I have done something with my memories this time. I have read books and asked questions. And in so doing I have touched the very face of evil. As I have researched the material for writing *Life on the Line*, I have at times thought that perhaps I could not endure any more. I have needed to feel clean again as I have read of little children put to death one by one in a white room with a geranium plant in the window. I have thanked God that there are still good men in the world when I have read of Raoul Wallenberg in Budapest and those German youths who called themselves the "White Rose" and gave their lives in the Resistance.

Above all, I have realized with chilling awareness that the days which led up to the atrocities in Hitler's Germany are not so different from these present days. We must remember, those of us who saw. We must begin to understand what we saw back then and put it together with what we see now. And we must tell the world what we discover.

In writing this book I have been reminded that as Christians "we wrestle not against flesh and blood, but against principalities, against powers, against the rulers of the darkness of this world, against spiritual wickedness in high places" (Ephesians 6:12). On a Sunday afternoon when I was particularly aware of the evil I was dealing with, I went back to the encouragement of certain books which have been old friends. Particularly in *Gold Cord*, by Amy Carmichael, I rediscovered some challenging thoughts that seemed to apply to the task before me:

Thou shalt have words,
But at this cost, that thou must first be burned,
Burned by red embers from a secret fire,
Scorched by fierce heats and withering winds that sweep
Through all thy being, carrying thee afar
From old delights. Doth not the ardent fire
Consume the mountain's heart before the flow
Of fervent lava? Wouldst thou easefully,
As from cool, pleasant fountains, flow in fire?[1]

And then a few pages later, in gentler words of encouragement:

At last a day came when the burden grew too heavy for me; and
then it was as though the tamarind trees about the house were
not tamarind, but olive, and under one of those trees our Lord
Jesus knelt, and He knelt alone. And I knew that this was His
burden, not mine. It was He who was asking me to share it with
Him, not I who was asking Him to share it with me. After that
there was only one thing to do: who that saw Him kneeling there
could turn away and forget? Who could have done anything but
go into the garden and kneel down beside Him under the olive
trees?[2]

The annihilation of the Jewish race was the goal of the
Holocaust. That was the Holocaust, and perhaps they are
right who say that that term should be reserved just for that
event. But there are implications from the Holocaust for us
today. What happened then evolved out of many factors
embedded in German society long before Hitler's day. Today,
many of those factors are present in American society, and
they threaten all of us and all of our children.

The Bible speaks of being as wise as serpents and as
gentle as doves. This is a day when great wisdom is needed,
and when great love and understanding are also needed
among people who sincerely disagree on the currently "hot"
issues of bioethics. Yet wisdom, love, and understanding
can only be applied to *knowledge*; they cannot be applied in a
vacuum. And so it is the purpose of this book to bring certain
facts as well as biblical principles to bear on the issues under

consideration. I do this as a family counselor who deals with people's pain on a daily basis, and as a Christian who tries to live by the principles of both the Old and New Testaments.

We are at a point where none of us can afford to say that topics like abortion and mercy killing are too troublesome to think about or too horrible to contemplate. We must deal with them, or the day will come when they will directly affect our own lives. Then we will regret that we did not get involved earlier.

When Lutheran pastor Martin Niemöller was lecturing across the United States after his release from the Nazi camps, he often closed with the following words:

> They came for the communists, but I wasn't a communist—so I didn't object;
>
> They came for the socialists, but I wasn't a socialist—so I didn't object;
>
> They came for the trade union leaders, but I wasn't a trade union leader—so I didn't object;
>
> They came for the Jews, but I wasn't a Jew—so I didn't object;
>
> Then they came for me—and there was no one left to object.[3]

Elizabeth Ruth Skoglund
Burbank, California
July 1989

ONE

" . . . And I Was Being So Good"

During World War II, "an eyewitness saw a mother and daughter at the head of a line going into the gas chambers of the concentration camp in Belzec, and he heard the child say, 'Mother, it's dark, it's so dark, and I was being so good.'"[1]

On April 15, 1945, units of the British Anti-Tank Regiment entered another concentration camp, this time at Bergen-Belsen. The very first British officer to enter the camp and view the ten thousand unburied bodies, many in a state of advanced decomposition, was ill-prepared for what he encountered. Wrote Derrick Sington:

> I had tried to visualize the interior of a concentration camp, but I had not imagined it like this. Nor had I imagined the strange simian throng, who crowded to the barbed wire fence surrounding the compounds, with their shaven heads and their obscene penitentiary suits, which were so dehumanizing. . . . We had been surrounded in Paris, embraced and thanked. . . . But the half-credulous cheers of these almost lost men, of these clowns in their terrible motley . . . impelled a stronger emotion and I had to fight back my tears.[2]

A few weeks after the liberation of Bergen-Belsen, the "official British gazette in the occupied zone wrote: 'The story of that greatest of all exhibitions of "man's inhumanity to man" which was Belsen concentration camp is known throughout the world.'"[3]

A friend of mine was released from Bergen-Belsen in late January 1945. For her, what these soldiers saw less than three months later was certainly not news. For her the dead bodies had been something to live with on a daily basis, as had the starvation diet, when they got it, of one liter of "soup," which consisted of water with a few turnips floating on top, and four centimeters of bread.

When I asked her what she remembered most from those teenage years in the camp, her first response was to tell of an incident which to this day evokes a visceral response in her when she thinks of it. It is a memory of a man riding a bicycle, following the inmates as they dragged their weary bodies to work. The man rode in among them, hitting one here and one there with his bike, just to scare them and hurt them. It was an experience of man's inhumanity to man which she could not forget.

Yet the Nazi Holocaust has not been the only example of man's inhumanity to man. It is just one of the most recent. Some day, like all the other atrocities of man's history, the story of the Holocaust may appear primarily in history books with an obscurity arising from the passage of the years. Obscure, not because it will become less true historically or less terrible, but because it will seem so long ago. It will be considered the barbarism of the past. Therein will lie the danger: that in its very obscurity, it will seem unreal—and it will be easy for people to forget that it could indeed happen again.

The atrocities of Hitler's Third Reich originated from philosophies and practices which extended back into the nineteenth century. However a major immediate factor was the poverty of Germany resulting in part from the Versailles Treaty ending World War I. Economic considerations, therefore, became involved in the killing. Then as today, how much society wants to pay in order to help the poor and the physically unfit determined policy. Robert Proctor writes of a document found in a castle which had been used as one of the six euthanasia institutions equipped with gas chambers, in which the following *savings* were cited as resulting from the involuntary euthanasia or murder of 70,273 persons:

Bread	4,781,339.72 kg.
Marmalade	239,067.02 kg.
Margarine	174,719.23 kg.
Schmalz	5,311.40 kg.
Coffee substitute	79,671.38 kg.
Sugar	185,952.86 kg.
Flour	156,952.86 kg.
Meats and sausage	653,516.96 kg.
Potatoes	19,754,325.27 kg.
Butter	50,458.49 kg.[4]

"The euthanasia operation had saved Germany an average of 88,543,980 reichsmarks per year and by the end of 1941, 93,521 hospital beds" were available due to the euthanasia program.[5]

Actually, gauging medical care by economic factors started at least in 1933, the first year of Nazi government, and then extended into the euthanasia program: German medical insurance companies paid 10 million reichsmarks *less* for the care of invalids in 1933 than in 1932 when Germany had been in the depths of the recession; many homes for the elderly were closed; the total number of working nurses taking care of the ill dropped from 111,700 in 1933 to 88,900 in 1934; the number of hospital and health care institutions decreased from 3,987 in 1931 to 3,219 in 1935; the number of hospital beds per 1,000 population went in the same time period from 5.7 to 4.5.[6]

At the time, a good summary statement of the official German attitude toward caring for the ill was: "From time immemorial, the nation has always eliminated the weak to make way for the healthy. A hard, but healthy and effective law to which we must once again give credence. The primary task of the physician is to discover for whom health care at government expense will be worth the cost."[7]

Similar Attitudes in America

During the time that millions were being slaughtered by the Nazis, the United States was not free from danger. Perhaps only the extremes of Hitler slowed down what could have been our own extremes and our own disregard for human life. In 1935, the French-American Nobel Prize winner Alexis Carrel, who ironically helped prepare the way for the transplant technology which has saved so many lives, suggested in his book *Man, the Unknown* that those who were criminal or insane should be "humanely and economically disposed of in small euthanasia institutions supplied with proper gases." In a 1938 speech to Harvard's Phi Beta Kappa chapter, W. G. Lennox stated that *saving* lives "adds a load to the back of society." He wanted physicians to recognize "the privilege of death for the congenitally mindless and for the incurable sick who wish to die; the boon of not being born for the unfit." And a 1937 Gallup Poll showed that 45 percent of the American population favored euthanasia for defective infants.[8] America was, indeed, well on her way then toward a disregard for human life; and she is well on her way once again.

Today, in a frightening manner, the idea of choosing who shall live and who shall die has been reappearing in both the United States and Europe. There is talk about rationing health care, limiting the amount of such care available to the poor or the chronically ill or the aged. According to a front-page article in the March 27, 1989 *New York Times*:

> The State of Oregon and Alameda County in California have become the first governments in the nation to plan explicit rationing of health care for the poor.
> In both places, agonizing choices are being made and lists drawn up, ranking medical procedures from the most effective

to the least, according to which save the most lives and improve the quality of life for the most people.[9]

The article goes on to say that officials in both Oregon and California . . .

hope to provide a model for rationing of care for the middle class by the Federal Government and by employers and insurance companies, which have been tightening restrictions on health coverage.[10]

In a May 15, 1989 article in *Time*, the comment is made that:

Many doctors readily admit that applicants for new high-tech operations have to pass a "green screen" or "wallet biopsy"— meaning those who can pay get first crack at the operations.[11]

According to *Time*, Dr. Marye L. Thomas, Alameda County's director of mental health, herself a member of a committee of experts designated to decide what treatments shall be available to the county's uninsured poor, commented:

As a physician, I was trained to give the best possible care to anyone, period. Back when I was in medical school, I never thought I would be discussing this.[12]

For us as in Nazi Germany there are also many factors which are preparing the way for the possibility of "medicalized" killing—the killing or assisted suicide of patients by doctors. We have talked about redefining death, for example, partly in order to justify the use of tissues and organs from anencephalic infants. We sometimes attempt to justify the possibility of medicalized killing when we refer to live human beings as "vegetables." There is talk about limiting the life span of the aged and terminating that of the terminally ill or defective.

If we were thrown into financial chaos, with the average person fighting for economic survival, we as a nation might be well on our way to denying basic health to large numbers of people—for even in our present prosperity we are approaching that point. Their treatment simply wouldn't fit our budget.

In 1988 an article in the *Los Angeles Times* stated:

> In findings that appear to reflect a significant degree of physician involvement in euthanasia, 79 California doctors claim they deliberately took the lives of terminal patients who asked to die, and 29 of them said they terminated the lives of at least three patients, according to a survey by the Hemlock Society, a national group that advocates euthanasia.[13]

In a recent article in the prestigious *New England Journal of Medicine*, the writers say that, "some of the practices that were controversial five years ago in the care of the dying patient have become accepted and routine." In its expansion of this statement the article claims later on that, "currently the courts are moving closer to the view that patients are entitled to be allowed to die, whether or not they are terminally ill or suffering." It claims that according to one public opinion poll, "68 percent of the respondents believed that people dying of an incurable, painful disease should be allowed to end their lives before the disease runs its course."[14]

As I write this morning, I have just read of the closing of another of many trauma centers in California. The reason given? Too many non-paying patients. People will die as a result of delayed treatment following an accident. Some will die who could have paid. And the next step may well be, as in the time of Nazi Germany, to decide more specifically who shall live and who shall die. The richest nation on earth may well decide that it can afford designer diapers, new cars as traditional sixteenth birthday presents, and dinners in Paris on special weekends, while not choosing to afford the care of the helpless and the ill, the aged and the maimed.

Moral Confusion

As I listen to those who consult me in my counseling office, repeatedly I am concerned about the confusion over the morality of these issues. Is it immoral for a childless couple to use a donor sperm in artificial insemination or a donor egg in in vitro fertilization, if that is the only way they can have a child? How far should a person go in avoiding pregnancy? Is it ever right to refuse medical treatment? At what point is it right to terminate on-going diagnostic procedures? What is the difference between terminating life and the prolonging of the dying process?

Such questions used to be asked by and debated among scholars and philosophers, not physicians, and certainly not by the layperson. Sometimes they were the topic of a science-fiction novel. Now, however, an ordinary citizen can't have a seriously ill relative without being asked whether or not the patient is a "no code"—a person for whom there will be no heroics performed. At death, or before death, relatives can be expected to be asked to immediately consent, or not consent, to the use of organs from the body of the loved one. This can be a rude shock to those not expecting it.

These problems, and many others like them, are relatively new to us. Before the revolution in medical technology, death was more easily defined. People who moved and made sounds were considered alive. If they stopped all movement and made no responses at all, they were considered dead. Doctors were there to save lives. Their goals were fixed: to heal and to comfort. Now their goals are not so clear. At some point they may feel that they are expected to be the executioner instead of the healer. After all, babies are sometimes allowed to die because they are considered aborted fetuses or products of conception, not babies. The terminally ill are at times aided in dying rather than helped to find meaning in living. And even if the actions taken are not as overt as these, at some point every physician is required to determine where life actually starts and where it ends.

If doctors are, at times, confused, the general population is at least equally confused. Young girls are encouraged by their friends one day to get an abortion, and shortly thereafter are told by the same friends that perhaps abortions are wrong. An adult child may decide that his parent is dead and order a respirator turned off, only to be told by his sister that he has just murdered their mother. These problems are being discussed, not just in doctors' offices, but in counseling offices, like my own, as well.

Among the most confusing and dangerous aspects of our new medical technology is that of *precedent*. What one chooses in one situation he or she might not want to choose in another. Allowing an overdose of morphine to terminate the life of a cancer patient who is in great pain and near death can easily lead, as we shall see later, to allowing the mercy killing, or suicide, of a healthy young person who is suffering from a bout of depression. Furthermore, medical guesses as to how soon someone will die, and whether or not the pain will continue to the same degree as before, are not always accurate. And in a controversial situation like the treatment of AIDS, while an AIDS patient might, in desperation, consent to euthanasia as his or her only solution, those with AIDS would certainly protest as a group, and rightly so, if all AIDS cases were automatically treated by so-called mercy killing. What might be considered by some to be a right in one situation could so easily turn into a violation of personal rights in another situation.

The right to voluntary euthanasia can never stay voluntary. For if when I am conscious I have the right to ask my physician to kill me, then, when I am unconscious, who will prevent someone else from killing me because they claim to know that is what I would have wanted? The transition from voluntary euthanasia to *involuntary* euthanasia is simple and natural—and inevitable. Most evil practices do not start out suddenly or obviously; they evolve—slowly and subtly.

The attempted annihilation of the Jewish race, before and during World War II, did not start out in practice as genocide.

A systematic process of genocide gradually evolved, but not before a precedent was established for killing in order to put people out of misery. The old, the infirm, the retarded, the maimed, among the Germans as well as the Jews—these were the first to be taken to "treatment centers." Mysterious letters would come to their relatives giving a variety of seemingly legitimate reasons for their deaths. Mercy killing came first, then genocide.

Christians Are Not Immune to These Issues

As we think about issues like abortion, euthanasia, and even genocide, Christians may be tempted to say, "none of those things will ever personally affect me." Just as the little girl at Belzec thought that because she had been good, bad things wouldn't happen to her, so some Christians feel that since they know God they are exempt from the human suffering that results from the sins of others. A good God will not allow pain. If euthanasia is legalized, we don't need to worry. We're Christians. Surely God will not let us be killed. If a law should be passed which prohibited the birth of children with Down's syndrome, we assume that somehow that law would never reach into our own household. But it might!

Both Scripture and the history of the church contradict the view that Christians don't suffer. All of Christ's disciples, with the exception of John, were executed for their beliefs. In the persecution which occurred within the first century after Christ's death, a law was passed "that no Christian once brought in before the tribunal, should be exempted from punishment without renouncing his religion." Furthermore, any disaster of nature, like an earthquake, pestilence, or famine, was attributed to the Christians.[15] Executions of the Christians ranged from beheading, burning at the stake, and stabbing, to broiling slowly over a fire and enduring all sorts of slow torture until, at the end, the execution was finalized with a quick stroke of the sword. Truly, they were "too good for this world" (Hebrews 11:38).

It is a common illusion among Christians today to feel that somehow we can demand something different. "Is not God a God of love?" we ask. Without listening for the answer of the still small voice within, and without consulting either our history books or our Bibles, we assume that, of course, a God of love will not let us suffer. Then when suffering enters our lives, we doubt ourselves and our faith as well as the goodness and even the existence of God himself. We not only endure the pain which has afflicted us, but we also suffer from our feeling that if God does not remove that pain according to our pleas then he, too, does not care or, perhaps, does not even exist. Sometimes we feel that while God may still exist, we ourselves must be sinning or we would not be suffering. It becomes a choice between denying God because of our pain, or deciding that while God still exists, he doesn't like us anymore.

"Why did my child die?" "Why is my son on drugs?" "Why is my wife (or husband) sleeping with someone else?" "Why me?" And, above all, "Why has God let this happen? I thought he was a God of love."

It has been said that the lives of the early Christians consisted of . . .

"persecutions above ground and prayer below ground." Their lives are expressed by the Coliseum (where they were often thrown to wild animals in order to amuse the crowd) and the catacombs. Beneath Rome are the excavations which we call the catacombs, which were at once temples and tombs. . . . There are some sixty catacombs near Rome, in which some six hundred miles of galleries have been traced, and these are not all. These galleries are about eight feet high and from three to five feet wide, containing on either side several rows of long, low, horizontal recesses, one above another like berths in a ship. In these the dead bodies were placed and the front closed, either by a single marble slab or several great tiles laid in mortar. On these slabs or tiles, epitaphs or symbols are graved or painted. Both pagans and Christians buried their dead in these catacombs.

When the Christian graves have been opened, the skeletons tell their own terrible tale. Heads are found severed from the body, ribs and shoulder blades are broken, bones are often calcined from fire.[16]

Did God not love these people who so faithfully served him and died for him? Unlike those of us who currently represent the body of Christ on this earth, those early Christians who endured such tremendous suffering did not seem to doubt the love of God because of that suffering. They did not question their own suffering for God when God's own Son, whom they had so recently known in the flesh on this earth, had suffered so visibly for them.

As we look at what was written on the walls of the catacombs, in contrast to an attitude of doubting God because of their suffering and "despite the awful story of persecution that we may read here, the inscriptions breathe forth peace and joy and triumph. Here are a few:

Here lies Marcia, put to rest in a dream of peace.

Lawrence to his sweetest son, borne away of angels.

Victorious in peace and in Christ.

Being called away, he went in peace."[17]

The hymn writer Isaac Watts expressed the concept of suffering as it relates to Christians in that remarkable hymn of the church, "Am I a Soldier of the Cross?" The second stanza asks:

Must I be carried to the skies
On flowery beds of ease,
While others fought to win the prize,
And sailed through bloody seas?

It is easy to sing such a hymn and not grasp its meaning. It is easy to read the Psalms for comfort and fail to question why, if God truly is in the business of automatically eradicating pain, David, who is called a man after God's own heart, suffered so much.

As a counselor who is in the business of improving the quality of people's lives, I would never advocate the cultivation of suffering for its own sake. While I would not argue with those who say that we grow through suffering, life seems to offer its own share of pain without our cultivating it. I totally concur with C. S. Lewis:

> When I think of pain—of anxiety that gnaws like fire and loneliness that spreads out like a desert, and the heartbreaking routine of monotonous misery, or again of dull aches that blacken our whole landscape or sudden nauseating pains that knock a man's heart out at one blow, of pains that seem already intolerable and then are suddenly increased, of infuriating scorpion-stinging pains that startle into maniacal movement a man who seemed half-dead with his previous tortures—it "quite o'ercrows my spirit." If I knew any way of escape, I would crawl through sewers to find it. But what is the good of telling you about my feelings? You know them already: they are the same as yours. I am not arguing that pain is not painful. Pain hurts. That is what the word means. I am only trying to show that the old Christian doctrine of being made "perfect through suffering" is not incredible. To prove it palatable is beyond my design.[18]

To predicate the love of God for any individual upon the absence of pain in his or her life, however, is to deny the example of Christ, the teaching of the Scriptures, and the example of the historical church. In a day when we hear talk of limiting health services for some, of euthanasia for others, of closing trauma centers, and of experimental medical projects which startle our sensitivities, we may well fear what could happen to us if we should become ill. This is particularly valid if we are aged or aging, or if we are poor or alone. Today many fear not receiving proper medical treatment. Others fear what could happen in the future.

Therein lies the glory of the love of God. We don't have to understand what God allows in order to rest in his love. For whatever we feel about what God should or should not do in order to qualify as a God of love, he remains a God of love. It is a great comfort to me personally to rest in that love and to know that ultimately he is in control. He will never stop loving me.

Sometimes God does, in his love, eradicate pain. Sometimes we are healed of physical affliction. Sometimes we are rescued from physical danger. God is still God, with all the power that goes into the very definition of God. God is still a God of miracles. Yet, very often, God does not eradicate our suffering, but rather, by his wonderful love, he carries us through.

God's Unconditional Love; Our Unconditional Faith

Perhaps the highest honor for a Christian is to be trusted to have unconditional faith in God's unconditional love. In one of my favorite poems, missionary Amy Carmichael wrote:

> Before the winds that blow do cease,
> Teach me to dwell within Thy calm;
> Before the pain has passed in peace,
> Give me, my God, to sing a psalm.[19]

Miss Carmichael's words are reminiscent of Job who, after answering those who claimed that his suffering was punishment for sin, declared: "Though he slay me, yet will I trust in him..." (Job 13:15), or, in G. Campbell Morgan's translation: "Though He slay me, yet will I wait for Him."[20] Any of us who have ever had to wait until the waiting, more than the thing we feared, became torture, will understand the added meaning of Morgan's translation.

But what is this love of God if it does not result in the eradication of pain? Where is this love if, in the middle of our confusion we cry out with our questions and do not hear a clear-cut answer? His love still comes as it did so long ago to those martyrs of the early church, not always in freedom from pain, but always in "enablement" through pain. The answers, too, do not always come in totality. Often, we are just led in part, as those who walk through deep fog and can only see what is in the immediate distance, each step that is ahead and no more. But, with God, we can be very sure of that one step. For God does not make mistakes.

Fifteen years ago, I wrote a magazine article on death; it was rejected by an editor who said that I did not have enough experience with death to write about it. She was correct. Almost no one I knew had ever died. Indeed, it was easy to have a false security and feel that death only happened to others.

Then my family all died in such rapid succession that I began to feel that, rather than never happening, death *always* happened to my family. I knew by memory the prices at the mortuary; I could close my eyes and envision the rows of different caskets in the display room. It got so that when we left the mortuary, the funeral director would say with genuineness that he hoped we would not be back soon. But we came back, in dwindling numbers. Then when the last relative, my aunt Lydia, was laid to rest, the funeral director—this time a new and younger man—looked around at the graves in surprise and asked, "Are all these from the same family?"

God had allowed my greatest childhood fear to come true. I remember the first time when, as a child, I looked into my mother's face and realized that no one else would ever be quite like her—and that someday she would die. Yet in these last fifteen years since members of my family first started to die, I have known the love of God in a way I had never experienced it before. His love has been tangible in a work

I enjoy, in friends who have been close as family, and, above all, in a sense of God's love and presence in my life which has shattered the sense of desolation I might have expected. God's love has made the difference in circumstances which might otherwise have been intolerable. He hasn't removed the circumstances, but he has helped me transcend them. God has not promised to make life easy, but he has promised to make it possible. And, much more than possible, for ultimately, in the middle of it all, there is always the love of God made tangible to us in some way. In the confusion of today's medical issues, we need this concept of the love of God more than ever. Of those students in the German Resistance who called themselves the White Rose, it was said that:

> Perhaps in ordinary times these young people would have remained unaffected by religious beliefs. . . . But the times were extraordinary. . . . Without a religious structure it was difficult; without God it was becoming impossible.[21]

Others have suffered and known the love of God. The hymn writer George Matheson was a young man in love. Then he was told the terrible news: he would be blind. To add blow to blow, his fiancée broke their engagement because of his impending blindness. In his brokenness, only the love of God prevailed, and he wrote the immortal words:

> O love that wilt not let me go,
> I rest my weary soul in thee;
> I give thee back the life I owe,
> That in thine ocean depths its flow
> May richer fuller be.

In words that cut across the lightness of our current superficiality regarding God's love, Matheson went on to conclude:

> O joy that seekest me through pain,
> I cannot close my heart to thee;

I trace the rainbow through the rain,
And feel the promise is not vain
That morn shall tearless be.

O cross that liftest up my head,
I dare not ask to hide from thee;
I lay in dust life's glory dead,
And from the ground there blossoms red
Life that shall endless be.

There is no god—be he any of the false gods men have sought through the ages or be he Jehovah God—who has eradicated the pain which exists on this earth. No god which man has sought after has made everyone happy on their terms. No god has given man all that he wants and evolved into something resembling a cosmic Santa Claus at Christmas time. If the eradication of pain is the qualification for being God then we have no God.

That is why people found God, and lost God, in the concentration camps. To some he became their solace, the only factor which made any sense. To others the camps obliterated any rational belief in God.

Today many incidents, both major and minor, are similar to those which led up to the Third Reich. A poor woman was told by a physician to walk on her foot until the huge piece of glass which was embedded in it "worked its way out." When questioned later about his actions, the physician replied: "I had too much to do that morning." A nurse commented, "She was just a cleaning woman." We are truly beginning to ration health care according to our fluctuating standards of who is worthy.

For many, while God is not someone to be denied, still he is on probation, particularly when the innocent suffer. He is God if he does it our way. In Jehovah God, however, we have God on his terms, not ours. On our terms, the memory of a little girl walking into Hitler's death camp with the words, "It's dark, it's so dark, and I was being so good," does not make sense if there is a God of love. Still, "though he slay me, yet will I trust in him" must be our answering cry in a world which often does not make sense. There must be unqualified faith in unqualified love. It is in faith in the unexplained love of Almighty God that we survive and go on dealing with the perplexing issues of the day, knowing that:

> For the present, we see things as if in a mirror, and are puzzled; but then we shall see them face to face. For the present the knowledge I gain is imperfect; but then I shall know fully, even as I am fully known. And so there remain Faith, Hope, Love—these three; and of these the greatest is Love (1 Corinthians 13:12-13, Weymouth).

TWO

A Decision to Love

A man who had been a prisoner in the Soviet Union's "Gulag" for some eighteen years and was used to the vicissitudes of prison life, the unexplained orders, the hopelessness, was abruptly put into a new cell. His new cell mate was the Swedish diplomat Raoul Wallenberg, who had saved so many Jewish people in Budapest at the end of World War II. The few hours he spent in Wallenberg's cell had been an obvious mistake, since Wallenberg was by that time kept from contact with other prisoners. And his placement in Wallenberg's cell was in itself just one additional disruption in prison routine. Yet in those few hours with Wallenberg there had been enough time for him to form an impression which he would not soon forget.

Almost a decade later, the prisoner was released. It was then that he went to Stockholm and told his story to Raoul Wallenberg's mother, who for years had been trying to effect the release of her son. He told how he and Wallenberg had communicated in prison sign language for the few hours they were together. But first Wallenberg, who was about to eat his daily bread ration, had broken it in half and silently handed a piece to his new cell mate. He was questioned about how he could be so sure that it was Wallenberg he was remembering, since the Soviets claimed that Wallenberg had died by that time. After all, he was reminded, considerable time had gone by—perhaps his memory was not accurate. The man replied that it was the first and the last time anyone in the Gulag had offered him a part of his precious bread ration. He could not forget such a person nor the date when they had met. He could not forget such love.

Raoul Wallenberg didn't know his new cell mate any more than he knew the thousands of Jews he pulled off of the trains headed for the camps. He surely couldn't have felt equally compelling love for each of these strangers. Yet his actions epitomized love in the truest sense of giving one's last crust and risking one's very life for another person. A great lesson to be learned from Raoul Wallenberg is the tremendous effect one man's decision to love can have on the lives of many.

As we come to the end of the twentieth century we are being given challenges to love which are unprecedented. In the areas of eugenics, abortion, euthanasia, alternative reproduction technology, and new medical treatments for a variety of diseases, there are often no fixed or consistent solutions. We are dependent, more than ever, on the guidance of God; and more than ever we are challenged to act in love toward those around us who may disagree, or who may, like us, be confused.

Le Chambon: City of Refuge

High in the mountains of France is a little town called Le Chambon. During World War II, the citizens of this village harbored roughly twenty-five hundred refugees from the Nazi terror. The village patterned itself after the Old Testament cities of refuge. In Deuteronomy 19:4 (RSV), we read that these cities were "the provision for the manslayer, who by fleeing there may save his life." Cities of refuge were set aside for those who accidentally killed someone. Once such a man reached a city of refuge, it was the responsibility of the residents of that city to protect his life. The villagers of Le Chambon reasoned that if a *manslayer* deserved such protection, certainly it was right to protect the totally innocent. They made their village a city of refuge, "lest innocent blood be shed" (Deuteronomy 19:10, RSV).

For the residents of Le Chambon, as with Wallenberg, there was not necessarily any surge of affection toward the strangers within their gates. They, too, didn't even know the people for whom they risked their lives. As time went by, personal feelings may have developed toward some. But essentially, like Raoul Wallenberg, the Chambonnais had simply made a decision to act in love.

Striking in her example of love as action was Magda Trocme, the wife of Pastor Andre Trocme, unspoken leader of the Resistance movement in Le Chambon. The little village had developed the reputation of being a "nest of Jews in Protestant country."[1] Trocme was once arrested for his activities and sympathies. The police arrived at dinner time, so Magda invited them to stay for dinner. When she was asked how she could be so decent as to eat with these men, how she could extend hospitality to them and forgive them, she replied:

> What are you talking about? It was dinner time: they were standing in my way; we were hungry. The food was ready. What do you mean by such foolish words as "forgiving" and "decent"?[2]

It was the same hospitable attitude she had shown when welcoming her first refugee from the Nazis:

> A German woman knocked at my door. It was the evening, and she said she was a German Jew, coming from northern France, that she was in danger, and that she had heard that in Le Chambon somebody could help her. Could she come into my house? I said, "Naturally, come in, come in."[3]

"Naturally, come in, come in" became the unwritten

slogan of Le Chambon. Those words represented the collective decision of a whole village to love. During the most violent years of World War II, the village of Le Chambon, high in the mountains of southern France, quietly saved people whom they didn't even know. Other villages in France were burned to the ground for less. Yet the little village survived and was called the safest place for Jewish people in all of Europe.

It is a principle of the Scriptures that as we act in love, and draw upon that One who is love and who dwells in us, more often than not, what started as an unemotional decision to love will change from actions alone into behavior which is motivated by *feelings* of love. Our responsibility is to choose to *act* in love. God's responsibility is to give the *feelings* of love.

Love defined by action can have a lasting impact in difficult situations. Albert Speer, architect of the Third Reich, and at one time one of Hitler's closest confidants, wrote movingly of those who guarded him at Spandau prison after his war crimes conviction:

During the next twenty years of my life, I was guarded in Spandau prison by nationals of the four powers against whom I had organized Hitler's war. Along with my six fellow prisoners, they were the only people I had close contact with. Through them I learned directly what the effects of my work had been. Many of them mourned loved ones who had died in the war— in particular, every one of the Soviet guards had lost some close relative, brother, or a father. Yet, not one of them bore a grudge toward me for my personal share in the tragedy; never did I hear words of recrimination. At the lowest ebb of my existence, in contact with these ordinary people, I encountered uncorrupted feelings of sympathy, helpfulness, human understanding, feelings that bypassed the prison rules. On the day before my appointment as minister of armaments and war production, I had encountered peasants in the Ukraine [an area in the Soviet Union which had suffered deeply under both Hitler and Stalin]— who had saved me from frostbite. At the time, I had been merely touched, without understanding. Now, after all was over, I once again was treated to examples of human kindness that transcended all enmity. And now, at last, I wanted to understand.[4]

Love Is *Action*

If it is our part to act in love and it is God whose love ultimately fills us, what then is the nature of this godly love? As we look around us today, at this time of transition into the twenty-first century, we see much that is called love. Weekend sexual affairs which are justified in the name of love; the aged sequestered in places where it is rationalized that "they will be with their own"; children shunted at whim from house to house in custody settlements ostensibly because they are "loved," but really at the convenience of the adults involved. All of these are just examples of our confusion about what love is.

In speaking of love in the New Testament, Paul says:

> Love is very patient, very kind. Love knows no jealousy; love makes no parade, gives itself no airs, is never rude, never selfish, never irritated, never resentful; love is never glad when others go wrong, love is gladdened by goodness, always slow to expose, always eager to believe the best, always hopeful, always patient. Love never disappears (1 Corinthians 13:4-8, Moffatt).

The New Testament uses two different Greek words for love which are applicable in this context. The noun *philia* means friendship, affinity toward, affection for. The other word *agape*, according to Dr. Alan Redpath, . . .

> means the actual absorption of every part of our being in one great passion. . . . This word has little to do with mere emotion; it indicates love which deliberately, by an act of will, chooses its object, and through thick or thin, regardless of the attractiveness of the object concerned, goes on loving continually, eternally. . . . It is always used when the will is involved rather than the emotions. That is why, in regard to the Christian's attitude to his enemy, this is the word which the Lord used: "thou shalt love [not phileo, "like," but agapao, "agonize over"] thine enemies.[5]

Yet the Bible goes further than just defining love. It says that without love we are nothing. Again, in 1 Corinthians 13 we read:

> If I can speak with the tongues of men and of angels, but am destitute of Love, I have but become a loud-sounding trumpet or a clanging cymbal. If I possess the gift of prophecy and am versed in all mysteries and all knowledge, and have such an absolute faith that I can remove mountains, but am destitute of Love, I am nothing. If I distribute all my possessions to the poor, and give up my body to be burned, but am destitute of Love, it profits me nothing (1 Corinthians 13:1-3, Weymouth).

Love is more than an emotion. Love is action. It is easy to tear down; it takes love—the biblical love which is *action*—to build up. There's an old saying that, "he has the right to criticize who has the heart to help." Don't criticize a homeless girl for getting an abortion, if you're not willing to help her find a home. Don't condemn someone who wants to die because of severe pain, unless you're willing to be a comforter to that person as he or she endures their pain. God save us from our own self-righteousness. It's not that we are to waver in what we believe but that we are to act out those beliefs in love. For in a practical sense it is the love of God lived out in the lives of those who know him which most of all reaches out and changes the lives of those around us—including our own brethren in Christ! People do not quickly forget love.

If love is action, then the ultimate challenge of that action, the final test of love, is to be willing to die. Henning von Trescow, who was one of Hitler's colonels who turned on him and tried to stop him, said to a comrade before he died:

> In a few hours time I shall stand before God, answering for my actions and for my omissions. I think I shall be able to uphold with a clear conscience all that I have done in the fight against Hitler.... The worth of a man is certain only if he is prepared to sacrifice his life for his convictions.[6]

Basing his words on a commitment to something even higher than a human fight against evil, Christ said: "I demand that you love each other as much as I love you. And here is how to measure it—the greatest love is shown when a person lays down his life for his friends" (John 15:13-14, TLB). One of the greatest challenges of the Christian life is to choose to act in love.

Acting in Truth and in Love

As much as a "black and white" approach to life can make some of us feel secure, we are moving into times when situations will arise involving legitimate grey areas. Nowhere is this more true than in the confusing issues of medical ethics. Some of us may be clear in our beliefs in areas like abortion and euthanasia, but God help us as Christians if, even when we are sure, we don't act in love toward those who disagree with us. And in those grey areas, where we dare not act as though we have all the answers, God help us if we act as though we do.

When God saw fit to take home all my earthly family with whom I had any real contact, he then gave me a person here and another there until I had a family once again, not one united by blood, but one united by caring, by friendship proven by the years and by a oneness in the body of Christ.

My aunt Lydia was the last one to die and so she was precious to me in a very special way. She had almost died in the car accident which took my mother's life. She endured the pain and the risk of three hip fractures. She had osteoporosis so badly that the X rays of her hip bones looked like transparent tissue paper. Yet at the age of eighty-nine she still walked.

On the evening of her death, she was different than she had been all of those other times when she had been so close to death. Each time before when she would say, "I think I'm going home to be with the Lord," it seemed right to disagree with her and encourage her to try to live. On this particular evening, as I approached her bed she opened her eyes and said decisively, "I'm dying." Just that. And I knew that she was right.

Yet a few minutes later, when a nurse came in and asked if I wanted a "no code" put on her chart, I panicked. I couldn't stop fighting for her to live, and I fervently wished for the old days when people just died because there was nothing else which medical science could do for them.

My immediate reaction was anger that I was the only one left to decide this. I longed for my family. I first decided I would solve my whole personal dilemma by simply not making a decision. But I knew that not to make a decision was to decide that she might be kept alive long after her time had come. But then wasn't that what medicine was supposed to do—keep people alive for as long as possible?

In my confusion, I went to a little coffee shop which had been a retreat for my friends and me as teenagers. In my booth, which was a small island in the middle of children screaming and adults rushing around, I thought and I prayed. I knew I didn't have much time. She would soon stop breathing and my decision would have been made for me. Without the "no code" they would pound and break those brittle bones with CPR, and perhaps put her on a respirator to breathe for her—a machine which at that time could not be turned off without a court order.

I find that often when I need God's guidance in the most complicated issues I get the simplest answers. With a deep sense of calm, suddenly I realized that I was not deciding whether or not my aunt should live—I was deciding whether or not to prolong her dying. She was dying. All man could do was painfully prolong that process. And so I decided not to intrude into God's timing for her death. Within seconds of conveying to the doctor my decision not to interfere, she stopped breathing and was with her Lord. It was in *his* time.

Such a decision was very difficult to make. There are

those who would say that she had already lived too long, that she should have died with that first hip fracture and made room for a younger generation. Some would say that total hip replacements at that age were too costly, especially since no one even expected her to walk after the third one. On the other hand, some would argue that every machine available should have been used to keep that frail body "alive." My decision was based on asking,"What is the will of God?"— not on trying to decide what was most loving. But as I carried out that decision, I acted in love toward her. I comforted her, I stayed with her.

The moral issues multiply as medical science advances. When should dialysis be used? When cardiac arrest has occurred, when should CPR be done and when is it too late to even attempt to start the heart beating again? To what extent should people avail themselves of chemotherapy? These and a thousand other questions have answers which are not always obvious or clear. The issues are not comfortingly "black and white." The answers are not clear cut.

In the middle of the confusion around us, and in spite of it, the Christian is commanded to love. Love is never offered in Scripture as a suggestion. It is always a command. "Love is ... always eager to believe the best, always hopeful, always patient. Love never disappears." How often we disappear when we disapprove of one another. Or worse still, how often we stay and disagree with absoluteness on questions which only God knows the answers to. How often we even enjoy disagreeing! Someday we Christians will have to stand before God regarding the correctness of our doctrine. Most of us realize that. But do we forget that some day we will also be judged for our lack of love? And all of our correctness will be as nothing if it was not enacted in love.

Because we are human we sometimes fail to allow God's love to show through us. But such is not God's ideal for his people. The other day I was feeling out of sorts with the world and with myself. The constant noise of construction across the street, the clanging of the ill-fixed gate outside of my window, the sudden escalating heat of late summer and the pressure of demands all combined to make me irritable. Later, as I was working on ideas for this chapter, I thought of the words in James 3:11-12, which speak of the Christian ideal of love:

> In a fountain, are fresh water and bitter sent forth from the same opening? Can a fig tree my brethren, yield olives, or a vine yield figs? No: and neither can salt water yield sweet (Weymouth).

In commenting on these verses, A. R. Fausset adds:

> The image is appropriate to the scene of the epistle, Palestine, wherein salt and bitter springs are found. Though "sweet" springs are sometimes found near, yet "sweet" and "bitter" (water) do not flow "at the same aperture." Grace can make the mouth that "sent forth the bitter" once, send forth the sweet.[7]

In other words, grace can change us.

Missionary Amy Carmichael's words on these verses are: "If a sudden jar can cause me to speak an impatient, unloving word, then I know nothing of Calvary love." She goes on to add in her footnote: "For a cup brimful of sweet water cannot spill even one drop of bitter water however suddenly jolted."[8]

While we will sometimes fail, if we are truly filled with the love of God, it will be the tendency of our lives to prevent injustice even when that injustice does not immediately touch us. If we are continually being filled with the love of God, such action will tend to be spontaneous, for we will be a fountain filled with sweet water. If I am of the belief that real humans are killed in abortion, I will act to stop abortions even if I am not pregnant. If I believe that euthanasia is wrong, I will act to prevent it before it affects me. I will care even when I am not personally involved.

I have been interested in the similarity at times between the scriptural definitions of love and of wisdom. For in those places where the Bible speaks of wisdom, it seems to emphasize loving entreaty, humility, and patience. In James 3:17

(Moffatt) we read: "The wisdom from above is first of all pure, then peaceable, forbearing, conciliatory, full of mercy and wholesome fruit, unambiguous, straightforward." *The Living Bible* says that wisdom "allows discussion and is willing to yield to others."

Along the same line of thinking, in chapter 38 of Job, Job exclaims "Who is this that darkeneth counsel by words without knowledge?" Job says that not only are these people making his pain more difficult to bear by their lack of love, but they are also making it harder for him to discern truth. According to Bible commentator Adam Clarke, Job said "Who art thou who pretendest to speak on the deep things of God, and the administration of his justice and providence, which thou canst not comprehend and leavest my counsels and designs the darker for thy explanation?"[9]

When we deal with people on issues of the day, if we do not do so in love we may only increase their pain. We may leave those whom we try to influence "darker" for our explanation. We may find ourselves becoming more anxious to prove our point than to meet the other person's need or even to defend the truth as we see it. For while a definition of truth cannot rest primarily on what is loving, truth, when expressed in a loving manner, will not be tempted toward the kind of error which arises out of an ego need to be different or to stand out regardless of truth.

Which One Gets Our Love?

The great error of so-called situation ethics was not that it emphasized love, but that it distorted love into an end in itself rather than focusing it back on God—and correct doctrine became less important as a result. As we approach the complex moral dilemmas of the twenty-first century, we cannot afford to base our ethics primarily on what is most loving. Today we face issues like the need of an unwed teenager to be free of an unwanted pregnancy balanced against the right of an unborn baby for a chance at life. If love is the basis for ethics, then which one gets our love? Obviously, in such a dilemma, we cannot with any consistency do as the proponents of situation ethics would suggest and base our moral position on love. That method never did work, and it will work even less effectively in the complex ethical issues with which we are being faced.

Our great example, Jesus Christ, did not hesitate to abrasively chase out the money changers in the temple. Righteousness must be upheld. With the woman caught in adultery, too, while he acted in infinite love and forgiveness, at the same time, he did not lower his standard of ethics, but rather told her to go and sin no more.

It is interesting that Joseph Fletcher, one of the most influential exponents of situation ethics, has according to a report in *Christianity Today* chosen to address the current bioethical dilemmas by "assessing" a patient's "personhood" in light of perceived quality of life rather than the simple biological fact of life. This concept of conditioning full personhood on the quality of life stands in contrast to the more traditional Christian principle asserting the sanctity of all human life regardless of its "quality."[10]

Christianity Today's report continues:

> According to Fletcher, a baby born with Down's syndrome may not be entitled to all the civil rights and spiritual dignity of personhood because of his or her impaired ability to reason and think.[11]

I am reminded of a psychologist friend who told me that when he worked in institutions, the most loving, sweet children to work with were those with Down's syndrome. It seems a little ironic that Fletcher, the man who would be willing to base his whole ethical system on love, denies personhood to at least some of these most loving of human beings.

In the Scriptures, we have an authoritative basis for a

concrete belief in God, and for making right ethical choices. We do not know all, nor shall we until eternity. But we know enough to have a basis for our beliefs and decisions. The authors of *Making Babies: The New Science and Ethics of Conception*, aptly state:

> Once we drop the idea that ethical knowledge is to be gained by special insight into the will of God, it ceases to be at all clear what is involved in being an expert in ethics. When it comes to ethical judgments, isn't everyone's opinion as good as anyone else's?[12]

Without God there is indeed no fixed ethical basis for dealing with the moral issues of our time.

Yet if truth cannot be based primarily on what is loving, still truth can become impotent if it is not exercised in love. "If I am versed in all mysteries and all knowledge . . . but am destitute of Love, I am nothing" (1 Corinthians 13:2, Weymouth). Once again the words of Paul call out with meaning for our time:

> For the present we see things as if in a mirror, and are puzzled; but then we shall see them face to face. For the present the knowledge I gain is imperfect; but then I shall know fully, even as I am fully known. And so there remain Faith, Hope, Love (1 Corinthians 13:12-13, Weymouth).

Without the love of God *to* us we cannot bear such times. Without the love of God *through* us, we will not be able to tolerate each other.

For those of us who know the love of God and do not act in its power, the result is particularly bitter for ourselves and for those around us. An unloving Christian is particularly unappealing. William Shakespeare wrote: "For sweetest things turn sourest by their deeds; Lilies that fester smell far worse than weeds."[13]

A new patient consulted me the other day and told me a moving story about his relationship with his physician. My patient, John, had been involved in a serious automobile accident, and so had required a long period of hospitalization and the extensive services of his orthopedic specialist. As he had watched this doctor function at different levels of stress and with a variety of hospital staff, he decided that the man had something he wanted. Under stress the physician still managed to be kind to everyone he encountered, and he had often extended himself beyond the call of duty. In those first few nights in the hospital, when no one could be sure that John would live or die, he would often wake up at odd hours of the night and find this doctor just checking to make sure his patient was okay.

After John was nearly recovered he went back for a monthly checkup.

"What makes you tick, doctor?" he asked curiously. "What turns you on? Because whatever it is, I've decided I want it. I've decided to be whatever you are, to join whatever you belong to."

"I'm a Christian," the physician responded simply. "I believe in Jesus Christ."

John became a Christian, and it was through his contact with this doctor that he finally ended up in my office. A man had acted in love to another human being whom he didn't even know. And because of that love, not only because of his great knowledge, he had saved not only his patient's body but had been instrumental in the saving of his eternal soul as well. This is what it means to be a instrument for the love of God. This is what happens when we make a decision to love.

THREE

Arsenal of Words

In my student days, I worked part time at a flower shop which provided flowers for funerals. We were required to ask questions about the deceased: the date of his or her death, the date of the service, where he or she would be interred. We were, above all else, forbidden to use words like, "dead," "buried," or "funeral." The idea was to be careful not to remind the customer of death, as if they could forget it now that they were buying flowers for a funeral! It was as if by changing the words about death, death itself could be forgotten.

One day an elderly lady called to order flowers for a funeral service. With my supervisor peering over my shoulder, I asked properly, "What is the name of the deceased?"

"What?" she replied.

Once again I asked, "What is the name of the deceased?"

"I just don't understand what you are saying," the lady replied with considerable irritation in her voice.

In a low but distinct voice I whispered, "Who died?"

"Oh," she responded cheerfully. "Is that what you wanted to know." And she went on to give me his name. Because of my supervisor's presence, we finished the conversation in the same cat-and-mouse fashion. "Where is he interred?" became "Where is he buried?" When was he deceased?"

changed into a hushed "When did he die?"

My experience with the use of words in the florist shop gave me my first conscious insight into their importance and also into how distortions of words can change their actual meaning.

Weapons for Good

Any student of history or literature can attest to the "weapon power" of words in major wars. Wars have often been fought as much with words as with guns.

Patrick Henry inflamed the American revolutionary cause with the words: "Is life so dear, or peace so sweet, as to be purchased at the price of chains and slavery? Forbid it, Almighty God!—I know not what course others may take; but as for me, give me liberty, or give me death!"[1]

In the same cause, Thomas Paine shamed his fellow men by challenging them to think of their children. Regarding what he saw as the inevitable break from England, he wrote:

> Not a man lives on the continent but fully believes that a separation must sometime or other finally take place, and a generous parent should have said, "If there must be trouble, let it be in my day, that my child may have peace."[2]

Few people would doubt the emotional impetus which a book like *Uncle Tom's Cabin*, by Harriet Beecher Stowe had on the American Civil War. The plight of Eliza and the mistreated but faithful Uncle Tom incited people against slavery; and, even though the Civil War was fought more to preserve the Union than to free the slaves, the emotional demand of the masses for freeing the slaves became an integral part of winning that war.

Words change us and our world; and when we use words as weapons, as a nation or as private citizens, the distortion of those words, or the invention of new words, sometimes becomes part of their effectiveness as weapons.

We generally reason that changes in meaning bring about changes in words. For example, with the advent of atomic warfare, we began to talk less about conventional weapons and words like *nuclear warhead* came into being. With the advent of space exploration, words like *launch pad* and *capsule* took on new meaning. The technology created the terminology.

In the area of medical ethics, however, the reverse seems to be occurring. As we change our words and create new ones, these new words in themselves help formulate our way of thinking. They become causal factors in our system of medical ethics rather than results of it. For example, when a physician says, "I'm just going to make her comfortable," it can mean just that. Or it can be an evasive statement which leaves the doctor free to treat without explanation. Under a dictatorship such a statement could be convenient and dangerous. It could mean: "I'll give her an overdose of morphine and put her out of her misery."

Sometimes when we don't want to face something we act as though it isn't there. I used a dog trainer to work with my dog, Horace. When Horace didn't like what the trainer was doing, he just turned his head and wouldn't look at him. Even food could not win him back. My other dog, Thackeray, who died a few years ago, used to bury his head in a pillow or blanket when he was afraid of the firecracker noise on the Fourth of July. He felt safe if his head was hidden. Now, turning your head or hiding it certainly doesn't make anyone safe. Indeed it may actually *decrease* the level of safety because you don't see what is coming next. So in the area of medical ethics, if we disguise the truth by word changes and even word distortions, we will not see what is coming next.

A Heritage of Evil Words

The people of pre-war Germany did not have any peculiar bent toward evil. With some cultural differences, they were just like you and me. Some entertain the idea that the Nazis were strange monsters who arose out of some bizarre and separate act of creation, in order to assure ourselves that we could never be like them. But even Adolf Hitler was conceived and born like everyone else. What happened in Germany was the result of a long-term form of brainwashing, originating in philosophies which had existed for generations and culminating in subtle uses of words which finally turned the tide toward a dramatic unleashing of evil.

Psychiatrist Viktor Frankl, a concentration camp survivor himself and a man with unusual insight into the Holocaust, wrote concerning the causes of the Holocaust:

> I am absolutely convinced that the gas chambers of Auschwitz, Treblinka, and Maidanek were ultimately prepared not in some ministry or other in Berlin, but rather at the desks and in the lecture halls of nihilistic scientists and philosophers.[3]

The philosophy of Friedrich Nietzsche and the personality of the musician Richard Wagner in the mid 1880s are examples of this long-term cultural preparation for the Holocaust. Hitler was deeply influenced by both men; it is said that he often listened to Wagner's music as he was making major military decisions.

In his masterpiece on the Third Reich, William Shirer wrote:

> I think no one who lived in the Third Reich could have failed to be impressed by Nietzsche's influence on it. His books might be full, as Santayana said, of "genial imbecility" and "boyish blasphemies." Yet, Nazi scribblers never tired of extolling him. Hitler often visited the Nietzsche museum in Weimar and publicized his veneration for the philosopher by posing for photographs of himself staring in rapture at the bust of the great man. . . .

Finally, there was Nietzsche's prophecy of the coming elite who would rule the world and from whom the superman would spring. In *The Will to Power*, he exclaims: "A daring and ruler race is building itself up. . . . The aim should be to prepare a transvaluation of values for a particularly strong kind of man, most highly gifted in intellect and will. This man and the elite around him will become the "lords of the earth."

Such rantings from one of Germany's most original minds must have struck a responsive chord in Hitler's littered mind. At any rate he appropriated them for his own—not only the thoughts but the philosopher's penchant for grotesque exaggeration, and often his very words. "Lords of the Earth" is a familiar expression in *Mein Kampf*. That in the end Hitler considered himself the superman of Nietzsche's prophecy can not be doubted.[4]

Shirer goes on to state: "'Whoever wants to understand National Socialist Germany must know Wagner,' Hitler used to say."[5] According to a *New Yorker* review of a collection of Wagner's letters, "The Master urges the ostracism, perhaps the actual eradication, of all European Jews." Indeed, in a letter to Franz Liszt of April 1851, Wagner wrote, "I harbored a long-suppressed resentment against this Jewish business, and this resentment is as necessary to my nature as gall is to the blood."[6]

Explains Shirer,

It was not his [Wagner's] political writings, however, but his towering operas, recalling so vividly the world of German antiquity with its heroic myths, its fighting pagan gods and heroes, its demons and dragons, its blood feuds and primitive tribal codes, its sense of destiny, of the splendor of love and life and the nobility of death, which inspired the myths of modern Germany and gave it a Germanic Weltanschauung which Hitler and the Nazis, with some justification, took over as their own.[7]

In the religious realm, too, it was unfortunate for the German people, the world, and especially God's chosen people the Jews that there were serious errors which paved the way for the atrocities which occurred. To quote once again from Shirer, who goes out of his way to state that he is a Protestant:

It is difficult to understand the behavior of most German Protestants in the first Nazi years unless one is aware of two things:
their history and the influence of Martin Luther. The great
founder of Protestantism was both a passionate anti-Semite and
a ferocious believer in absolute obedience to political authority.
He wanted Germany rid of the Jews and when they were sent
away he advised that they be deprived of "all their cash and
jewels and silver and gold" and, furthermore, "that their syna-
gogues or schools be set on fire, that their houses be broken up
and destroyed . . . and they be put under a roof or stable, like the
gypsies . . . in misery and captivity as they incessantly lament
and complain to God about us."—advice that was literally
followed four centuries later by Hitler, Goering and Himmler.[8]

Earlier in his life Luther had expressed an opposite point
of view. Of those who mistreated Jewish people, he had said:
"By this tyrannical attitude of theirs these godless people,
who are Christians in name only, are inflicting no light injury
on the Christian name as well as Christian people."[9] On
another occasion he complained of church leaders who:

> . . . have hitherto treated the Jews in such a way that whoever was
> a good Christian was almost tempted to turn Jew. If I had been
> a Jew and had seen such boors and brutes control and teach the
> Christian faith, I would rather have become a sow than a
> Christian: for Jews were treated as if they were dogs and not
> human beings.[10]

Later, however, when he wrote *Von den Juden und ihren
Lugen (About the Jews and Their Lies)*, his writing had become
distinctly anti-Semitic. One Luther scholar explains: "He
had become disillusioned. The Jews did not welcome the
gospel when it was preached to them in apostolic purity. . . .
Therefore Luther decided to cover the matter thoroughly,"[11]
and, one might add, abusively, without a display of love!

In *Here I Stand, A Life of Martin Luther*, Roland Bainton
explains the two extremes more completely. According to
Bainton, Luther felt that, by eliminating the abuses toward
the Jews, they could be converted. And when that didn't
happen, when, indeed, certain rabbis even tried to convert

Luther to Judaism, he struck out in words of vengeance against them:

> One could wish that Luther had died before ever this tract was written. Yet one must be clear as to what he was recommending and why. His position was entirely religious and in no respect racial. The supreme sin for him was the persistent rejection of God's revelation of himself in Christ.... Luther justified himself by appealing to the ire of Jehovah against those who go awhoring after other gods ... but he might have recalled that Scripture itself discountenances human imitation of the divine vengeance.[12]

It has been difficult for me, an evangelical Christian inspired daily by a plaque which hangs on my bedroom wall and is inscribed with words of Luther, to write of his opposition to God's chosen people. Yet his thinking ironically provided an impetus for the atrocities of Nazi Germany as well as for the great positive changes of the Reformation. Satan must have taken a peculiar joy in watching a man who had been used so greatly for good now being used so greatly for evil. Ironically, the greatness of his work for God in the Reformation may have made him particularly vulnerable to Satan's attack. Luther's life should be a stern warning to all of us of the danger of allowing prejudice into our thinking at all. Such potential for evil on the part of God's saints is very humbling indeed!

Dangerous Good-Sounding Words

To a nation which had grown up viewing Jewish people as their enemies, it was easy for Germans to be taken in by what the Nazis were doing, especially as those deeds began to be couched in euphemisms which blunted their true meaning and made the proposed deeds seem at least less ominous than they really were.

The word euphemism comes from Greek roots meaning

"good sound." And euphemisms can, in truth, be used for good purposes. They can soften a harsh reality or even, in select circumstances, alter truth so that a person's feelings can be spared. The night my mother died, my aunt Lydia, who had sustained serious injuries in the same car accident, was in a semi-private hospital room with my mother. When my mother suddenly died, Aunt Lydia was quickly moved into a private room. My prayer that August evening was that God would not take my mother and my aunt at the same time.

With that kind of emotion, I went into my aunt's room.

"Where's Betty?" were her first words. I could tell from the way she asked the question that she didn't know her sister had died. It was essential because of her precarious condition that she not know. Euphemisms were in order.

"She's in a room down the hall," I replied.

"What's happening?" she continued.

"They're taking care of her," I replied with technical honesty but not total truth. "She's okay now," I continued euphemistically, knowing that, since she was with her Lord, she was better off than any of us!

"You're like an angel from heaven," my aunt murmured sleepily as she drifted off to the restoration of sleep. A few days later my aunt asked, "What's happened to Betty? I can handle it now." And so I told her.

Euphemisms can be used for good; but more often than not they are used to blunt the appearance of evil. And they become actual enablers of evil. They were used during the Third Reich to keep the German people and the world from facing the reality of what was happening to the Jews, and they are used today with alarming success in various areas of bioethics. Jews were "relocated" rather than sent to concentration camps. Genocide was called the "final solution." When at last the euphemisms had totally eroded the image of the Jew, what had been said euphemistically could be freely stated. This was most effectively declared by a judge in an article published in October 1938, in the journal *Deutsche*

Justiz (German Justice):

> The Jew is not a human being. He is an appearance of putrescence. Just as the fission fungus cannot permeate wood until it is rotting, so the Jew was able to creep into the German people, to bring on disaster, only after the German nation, weakened by the loss of blood in the Thirty Years War, had begun to rot from within.[13]

"The Jew is not a human being." To be declared non-human: this is to open the door to a killing process which is then made possible with less conflict of conscience. In a strikingly similar way, to call an unborn child an "embryo" or a "fetus" results in a dehumanization of unborn human life which then enables abortions to become acceptable. When the word changes, the philosophy changes, and when the philosophy changes, the action changes.

"Quality" of Life

Today the road to euthanasia, or so-called mercy killing, is a similar one, which, along with abortion, derives part of its' justification from a euphemism like "quality of life." In order to justify either euthanasia or abortion, the term "quality of life" must replace the older concept of "sanctity of life."

"Sanctity of life" refers to life as sacred in and of itself. The term involves an unqualified respect for human life. The fact that God holds the timing and circumstances of our lives in his hands is a biblical principle which is consistent with a sanctity-of-life point of view.

The *Encyclopedia of Bioethics*, often called the "bible" of bioethics, includes a lengthy discussion of the quality-of-life viewpoint. According to this standard, says the *Encyclopedia, . . .*

> life need not be sustained or may be directly terminated if the quality of life is not satisfactory. The ethical question is: What principles should govern the use of a quality-of-life concept in a

possible justification for the termination or continuation of human life, especially the life of the defective, diseased, comatose, seriously ill, or dying patient of any age?[14]

The *Encyclopedia* goes on to draw from the thoughts of Joseph Fletcher in support of this viewpoint:

Human life has no value unless it produces personal well-being, here interpreted as human happiness for the largest number of people. The direct or indirect killing of a human is good whenever it is justified by this highest value or whenever the desirable consequences outweigh any disvalue in the action, according to a cost-benefit analysis.[15]

Continuing its presentation of Fletcher's views, the *Encyclopedia* observes that:

Fletcher's minimal "humanhood" criteria are associated with rational function; they include neocortical function (which is a prerequisite to the others), intelligence (humans scoring below 40 IQ are questionably persons, and below the 20 mark they are not persons), communication, and other qualities. Accessory qualities (he calls them "optimal criteria"), which contribute to an individual's better well-being, include curiosity, balance of rationality and feeling, and idiosyncrasy. . . . If the humanhood qualities are lacking, there is no moral offense in terminating a human life; if they are present, the moral value of preserving or terminating a life is known only by a utilitarian assessment of the needs of all those affected in each situation.[16]

In essence, according to the definition of quality of life, man, not God, determines and defines the value—or lack of value—of any given human life. Furthermore, even if a life has some value, the needs of others, the subjective factor of happiness, and even economics determine whether or not that life shall continue. Imagine, for example, a middle-class family with two sets of elderly parents to care for as well as three college age or near college age children to educate. They are having financial trouble because of all these responsibilities; furthermore, two of the elderly parents are discontented with their lives and require expensive medication and frequent attention. In such a situation, should euthanasia be considered? Such could have been the case for the multiply handicapped Helen Keller, before she had had a chance to prove the worth of her existence. Such could be the case for many handicapped or just life-weary people.

Just as abortion has become a sloppy form of birth control, so euthanasia could become, under the quality-of-life criteria, a fast solution for many problems ranging from financial hardship to a discontent with life itself. One thing we can be sure of is that, once man gives himself the authority to decide when others should live or die, the limits of that authority will never stop with mere alleviation of pain for the terminally ill. As we have seen, what begins as voluntary euthanasia will always become *involuntary* euthanasia—where the decision to die is made *for* you. To view it otherwise is to be naive.

Unworthy of Life?

In a chilling parallel to the term "quality of life," the Nazis had another favorite phrase which was more honest and blunt: *"lebensunwertes leben,"* which translates as "life unworthy of life." The killing machine of the Third Reich progressed from forced sterilization, through various stages of euthanasia, to actual genocide, all based on determinations that certain lives were not worthy to continue.

In discussing which lives should be thus deemed unworthy, Hitler proclaimed:

> The volkisch state must see to it that only the healthy beget children. . . . Here the state must act as the guardian of a millennial future. . . . It must declare unfit for propagation all who are in any way visibly sick or who have inherited a disease and can therefore pass it on.[17]

This definition of "life unworthy of life" continued to be a definitive basis, in Germany, for euthanasia and genocide as well as for forced sterilization.

Ironically, at the time when forced sterilization was begun in Germany, some German scientists were looking to America as the trend-setter in that practice. For whereas Germany's Weimar Constitution forbade the "infliction of bodily alterations on human beings," in the United States there were (as we shall see later in more detail) sterilization laws in existence, as well as laws which forbade the marriage of the mentally retarded and those of different races. Indeed, because of our "progress" in such areas at that time, a German physician-geneticist berated his own country's backwardness in comparison with the United States; he was "convinced that 'the next round in the thousand-year fight for the life of the Nordic race will probably be fought in America.'"[18] As we consider the similarities between our quest for what we call the right quality of life, and the Nazis' term life unworthy of life, it is vital that we consider whether we are heading toward our own "pure race" goal, however we may uniquely define such purity.

Once Hitler came to power in 1933, strict sterilization laws were put into effect. These were the first step in insuring the elimination of those with life unworthy of life. At first, some of those included were people with congenital feeblemindedness, schizophrenia, manic depression, hereditary blindness or deafness—and even alcoholism! The list broadened, of course, until eventually the entire Jewish race was deemed unworthy of life.

Quickly, too, the *method* of purifying the race was extended from merely preventing the conception of those with life unworthy of life to killing those already alive, until an estimate of one million people to be killed was published in a Nazi magazine in 1939.[19] The killing went beyond the individual's right to die. The state itself could legally kill, whether or not the person himself wanted to live. Yet curiously enough, the killing task always remained the task of the physician. It was always medicalized killing.

As early as 1920, two German scholars, Karl Binding and Alfred Hoche, had written a book titled *The Permission to Destroy Life Unworthy of Life*, in defense of such "medicalized" killing. Commenting on that book, Robert Lifton says:

> The book included as "unworthy life" not only the incurably ill but large segments of the mentally ill, the feebleminded, and retarded and deformed children. More than that, the authors professionalized and medicalized the entire concept. And they stressed the *therapeutic* goal of that concept: destroying life unworthy of life is "purely a healing treatment" and a "healing work."[20]

Hoche further emphasized that the killing was compassionate. He described these people as "empty shells of human beings." Says Lifton, "He was saying that these people are already dead."[21] Once again words were used to distort and thus legitimize what was being done. The evil was facilitated by euphemisms.

So the arguments raged in the Third Reich, and so they persist today. Those with "life unworthy of life" or those without "quality of life" should move over and make room for superior human beings. According to the proponents of these doctrines, when life *seems* to lose its meaning, when the body doesn't function as well as it used to, when the brain functions at a level of intelligence which is no longer "productive" by someone else's definition, and when it costs too much to keep one alive, then that person of compassion and healing, the family doctor, should simply put his patient to sleep. All of this because we change from a sanctity-of-life to a quality-of-life standard.

Best-selling Author; Lover of Trees

Words can be dangerous weapons for evil or vital weapons for truth. Just as the well sharpened sword can be used to destroy the enemy and protect the innocent, or that same sword can be the murder weapon of a midnight attacker of innocent victims, so words can be used for good or evil. And one of the most subtle uses of words is the euphemism, where meanings become distorted so that what looks like one thing becomes another. Evil can begin to look good. Nowhere has this happened more, in our time, than with the phrase quality of life.

Christopher Nolan is a young man in Dublin, Ireland. Brain-damaged at birth and therefore unable to speak or use his limbs, he has yet become a best-selling author. Much of his communication is through his eyes, while he types his books by the help of a pointer attached to his forehead.

In his thinly-disguised autobiographical book, *Under the Eye of the Clock*, Nolan writes in his unique style:

> The future for babies like him never looked more promising, but now society frowns upon giving spastic babies a right to life. Now they threatened to abort babies like him, to detect in advance their handicapped state, to burrow through the womb and label them for death, to baffle their mothers with fear for their coming, and yet, the spastic baby would ever be the soul which would never kill, maim, creed [sic] falsehood, or hate brotherhood. Why then does society fear the crippled child, wondered Joseph out loud, and why does it hail the able-bodied child and crow over what may in time become potential executioner?[22]

Christopher Nolan never ceases to marvel at the sacrifices his family has made for him. He has felt acutely the pain of his handicap and its isolation. Yet, as he puts it, "Banished dreams always healed in the presence of God."[23] And, "fenced in on all sides he heard things he was never meant to hear and he saw things he was never meant to see."[24] He was "harassed but not cheated—hurt but desperate to survive."[25] ". . . if computer science can give me a voice, then everyone else who is similarly affected stands a chance of being freed."[26]

As far back as 1973, *The New England Journal of Medicine*

reported that "of 299 consecutive deaths occurring in a special-care nursery, 43 (14 percent) were related to withholding treatment" because of a decision "that prognosis for meaningful life was extremely poor or hopeless."[27] While some of those babies may have been dying and, therefore, may not have warranted intervention which could only prolong that process and its pain, some may have been potential Christopher Nolans.

An elderly man had come home from his daily visit to his wife, who had been placed in a convalescent home with Alzheimer's disease.... As he sat down wearily in a chair, a close friend asked him why he bothered to visit so regularly. "She doesn't even know you're there," the friend concluded.

Thoughtfully the man gave his answer: "Sometimes maybe she does know I'm there," he said slowly:

> But it's more than that. More often than not I go for me. There's a big tree right outside of her window. We both always loved trees. Sometimes we would spend our vacations by going to the Redwoods, and we would continually marvel at the miracle of a tree. Now there are times when we sit in silence with our arms around each other and just look at that tree outside of her window. It seems to quiet her, and I can't tell you how much it comforts me. I feel like I have a little of her back. I feel like I'm also learning slowly how to give her up. In a way I'm grieving as I watch her slip further and further away from me. It's easier for me that way than all at once.

Quality of life? I don't think she would qualify by any of the current definitions. Life unworthy of life? By the standards of many, yes. Except, of course, in the opinion of God, who for some reason known to him alone still keeps her alive. Even on earth, in at least one man's mind she does have value. And when she really leaves him, this man will feel her loss as surely as any other man who experiences the death of a spouse. To him, and to God, she is still a human being; and no arsenal of words or opinions of man can change that fact.

FOUR

Enabling Evil

Medicine and literature held equal appeal to me as a student, both in high school and in the early days of my university life. Since they were such divergent interests, I spent a number of years literally running from one end of the campus to the other, taking Puritan Literature or Shakespeare one hour and Invertebrate Zoology the next. Because becoming a physician was a possible vocational goal, and because I loved studying in the biological sciences, performing dissections became mandatory.

"Frog," "blood," "guts,": such words signaled to my brain situations I was not good at handling. Watching a bull maul a man in a rodeo had been one of the greatest traumas of my childhood, and I had run away from the scene when a neighbor killed a chicken. I couldn't look at car accidents without feeling sick, and, as I approached adulthood, I worried about the day when I would encounter an accident where my help might be required.

When I walked into my first laboratory assignment where dissection was required, I was in high school and the specimen was only an earthworm. The problem was, I didn't like to even touch worms, much less cut one up. The word "worm," like frog, signaled a reaction of revulsion.

The second dissection came later with a frog, which was

even worse. Not only was I squeamish about frogs, but here was a creature with a whole lot more insides to dissect than any earthworm! A sense of defeat filled my being as I approached the huge jar of plump frogs soaking in formaldehyde. I couldn't even pick the thing up, much less cut into it. It was then that I realized I had to talk myself into a different mind-set. I couldn't readily change my gut reactions to "frog." But I could cease to see this creature primarily as a once-living creature.

The frog became to me a "frog-specimen." Cutting into it became an "experiment." The "innards" became internal organs which were talked about in terms of a "pump which forced life sustaining fluid throughout the body." "Guts" became an "intestine" or a "stomach." My language became clinical rather than personal. Having lost my focus on "frog," I became immersed in the miracle of the circulatory system, and marvelled at the similarity of design between that system as I saw it in this specimen and the one which God has given to us humans.

The frogs in the lab became permanently frog-specimens, not frogs. Other frogs still lived in ponds and jumped, and I still kept my distance from them. The "frog-specimen" became safe while my view of "frog" in general remained unchanged. The words frog and frog-specimen each became a signpost pointing to a different meaning. "Frog" meant a messy, living creature which I could not cope with. Calling a frog a frog-specimen detached me from any personal reactions, thereby enabling me to dissect them.

Signposts signal a larger meaning by the use of symbolic words. "Fifty seems to indicate the beginning of "over-the-hill" jokes and cosmetic surgery. "Teenager" has come to include a sort of caricature of a person who is unmanageable, selfish, loud, and in general difficult. Sometimes one wonders if most kids wouldn't grow up a lot easier if they were not expected to live up to the image of "teenager." Other words like "menopause," "middle-aged," "intellectual," "liberal," and "conservative," or phrases like "the terrible twos," all signal meanings far beyond the scope of one word. They have lost their precision of meaning, and they have an emotional charge to them which exceeds the simple definition of a word. They create fear or elation or commitment, depending on individual interpretation. They have become more than just words; they have become a catalyst for a whole series of visceral reactions. They are signposts which point in a general direction.

"Signposts" Enable Evil Actions

Words as signposts enable us to tolerate situations we don't want to face. They blunt or deaden the impact of the word they point to. The florist shop which used words like deceased instead of dead, or interred instead of buried, was trying to soften the reality of death. Likewise elderly people become "senior citizens," and children who are hard to place in adoptions, or mentally retarded children in the classroom, are all called "special."

During the Nuremberg trials after World War II, it was observed that the evidence presented against the defendants seemed to have little impact on them. These were Hitler's top henchmen, responsible for many of the atrocities of the Third Reich. Yet they remained relatively impassive. A verbatim diary which was kept of these reactions suggests a possible explanation, involving the careful use of those words which would buffer the defendants from directly confronting the reality of what they had really done. The words were signposts:

> They seldom used such words as "murder," "torture," "starvation." They slithered away from the specific and hid in euphemisms, cloaking facts in vagueness: "such things," "those horrors." The defendants had always avoided the nasty words. All their documents spoke not of their hatred and jealousy or ideological ambitions for the Jews, but of "the Jewish Problem" (just as they never wrote of ambitions or even fears when dealing

with Poland, but of "the Polish Problem")....From this starting point they could bypass the need to say "we want to get rid of the Jews" or "we want to invade Poland" and instead say "the Jewish problem must be solved" or "the Polish problem cannot be allowed to continue" (faced with a problem after all it is only right and proper to try to solve it). It was a simple linguistic dodge to skirt around the harsh black and white of "we have decided to kill all Jews" or "we will invade Poland," and to resort to the more euphonious "it has been decided to implement the Final Solution" or "steps are to be taken to secure Germany against the Polish menace."

[They] continued to use the vocabulary which had always saved them from the trouble of thinking.[1]

As in the Holocaust, so in the realm of the current bioethical controversy, words used as signposts often become clearcut enablers of behavior. Without at this point getting into the right or wrong of abortion, it provides good examples of signposts as enablers. A word like "fetus" can dull the impact of abortion; even people who do believe that life starts at conception can get used to the idea of killing a human life . . . by using a signpost like "terminating a pregnancy" or "aborting a fetus." Words like "murder" or "kill" are not as easy to deal with for they clarify reality. However, once a phrase like "terminating a pregnancy" has been used long enough, it has a desensitizing effect so that harsher words like "kill" are no longer disturbing.

In my counseling office, women who want to discuss getting an abortion used to come in and agonize over whether or not this "fetus" inside them was really a baby. A lot of debate went into when life started. People had trouble with abortion if they viewed the unborn life as a human being.

Today I don't hear that as much. Now women often say things like, "I know that this baby is a human being, but it's just not a good time for me to have a baby." They feel uncomfortable in killing what they now view as a baby, but not so uncomfortable that they change their minds about the abortion. The use of the word fetus for so many years, which enabled women to question the humanness of the life they were about to abort, has brought us to the point where we really aren't too concerned about when life starts. We have become used to discarding, not only what we view as "bits of protoplasm," but also what we view as actual human life. The signposts have shaped our way of thinking, rather than merely indicating what that thinking is. They have blunted the emotional impact of what is happening.

"Forward-Reversing"

Signposts enable a human being to completely reverse his or her normal pattern of behavior without facing the fact that it is a reversal. I will refer to this process as "forward-reversing," for it involves changing the direction of behavior while maintaining the illusion of continuing in the same direction. A trivial example of "forward-reversing," comes from my experience as a public speaker. Generally I don't like to do public speaking. But I do like to teach and appear on talk shows. I find both the give and take of conversation and the challenge of instruction to be stimulating. When I need to do straight public speaking I am enabled to do it if I can view it as a teaching or question-and-answer situation. I still "don't do public speaking." I "discuss" or "teach." I change the meaning of what I am doing by changing the words. I *never* call it "giving a speech."

Forward-reversing can sometimes simply enable us to do what we must do. When President John Kennedy was assassinated in Dallas, the newscasters of that day were as emotionally shocked as anyone else but they were not as free to break down and cry or to indulge their feelings. As the first words of Kennedy's death came through the news service from two priests at Parkland Hospital, the newscaster who announced that the President had indeed died started to break down. His normal reactions as a human being and as a citizen of the United States were at first automatic. He quickly reversed himself, however, and as he confronted a whole nation he became the outwardly controlled news-caster. A citizen manifesting uncontrolled grief and a news-caster reporting news were not at that time compatible with each other. For the moment human reactions were mini-mized and reporting the news became the focus. He for-ward-reversed from the direction of private citizen to that of public figure.

All of us use forward-reversing. But unfortunately the results are not always as innocent as my example of public speaking nor as moral and yet practical as the example of the newscaster. For example, a man with a sick child who is a good husband and father, who values integrity in his rela-tionships with his wife and friends, may go to work and embezzle funds. This is a forward-reversal of his behavior outside the market place. But in his mind, since his child needs surgery, embezzling funds is an extension of being a good father. Dishonesty becomes less the focus than "good father." And "good father" becomes the consistent factor in his life. "Good father" is the signpost which enables the forward-reversal.

Psychoanalysts have used the term "splitting" or "dou-bling" to describe the same sort of thinking. Lifton says:

> The key to understanding how Nazi doctors came to do the work of Auschwitz is the psychological principle I call "dou-bling"; the division of the self into two functioning wholes, so that a part-self acts as an entire self.[2]

I find it slightly easier to understand the enablement of evil, and for that matter the enablement of good, in terms of what I have called forward-reversing, where rather than dealing with "two functioning wholes" we deal with one whole which, under the deception of going straight ahead, turns and goes in the opposite direction.

A hospital which deals in abortions as well as intensive care for the newborn is, in my mind, a place where such forward-reversing will occur. In such a hospital a young physician doing his rounds noticed a baby lying on a counter, unobserved, uncared for. The infant had been aborted a few hours previously but had not conveniently died. The physician was on his way to the neo-natal intensive care unit where babies as small or smaller were being given all the care possible in order to save their lives. Unable to forward-reverse effectively and leave this child to die while he saved others who were in a worse condition, he grabbed the baby and brought it to the other end of the hall for help.

Joseph Mengele, camp doctor at Auschwitz, known to many as the "Angel of Death," was a master at forward-reversing in order to accomplish blatant evil. Allowing himself the consistency of remaining the compassionate physician in order to justify the forward-reversal from doctor-healer to doctor-killer, Mengele explained:

> When a Jewish child is born, or when a woman comes to the camp with a child already, I don't know what to do with the child. I can't set the child free because there are no longer any Jews who live in freedom. I can't let the child stay in the camp because there are no facilities in the camp that would enable the child to develop normally. It would not be humanitarian to send a child to the ovens without permitting the mother to be there to witness the child's death. That is why I send the mother and child to the gas ovens together.[3]

It was these kinds of rationalizations which enabled the forward-reversals in Mengele, where he played with children and even had his favorites, and then suddenly, when he had finished experimenting with them, killed them. His consistent signposts were the purification of race and the curing of the cancer which had intruded upon that race, the Jews. Above all, he was enabled by the signpost of "non-human," as it applied to the Jewish race. Thus he could forward-reverse back and forth, healer and killer, and be consistent with himself. Mengele is perhaps one of the best examples of how evil can be enabled by words which are used as signposts and by the process of forward-reversing.

There were many such enablers for the doctors of the Third Reich, for Hitler maintained that the killing process should always remain medicalized killing. Euthanasia or mercy killing came under the heading of preventative medicine; and Jewish people who were suspected of spreading an epidemic had to be killed for the good of the whole. The disease became synonymous with the person and the preventative method was not their cure but their eradication.

Prevention Then and Now

The emphasis on preventative medicine in the Third Reich bears a striking resemblance to our own emphasis on an approach to medicine which seems so positive and, in truth, has much value. To treat the whole man, to emphasize good nutrition and ample exercise are in themselves helpful. The Nazis, like us, discouraged the use of tobacco as well as alcoholic beverages and emphasized in their place fruit juices and mineral water. Indeed . . .

> medical leaders in the Nazi government commonly spoke of the need to reorient medicine from an emphasis on curing ailments to an emphasis on preventing them. The racial hygiene program was itself conceived along these lines: racial hygiene was intended to provide long-term preventive care for the human genetic material.[4]

Gerhard Wagner, who was "Führer of the Nazi Physicians' League," among other impressive titles, stated that,

> It is not enough for the National Socialist health policymaker to eradicate already existing diseases; he must avoid and prevent them. The healthiest people is not that which possesses the best, or the greatest number of hospitals, but rather that which needs the fewest.[5]

To the Nazis the focus was on health, but mainly because good health related to the preservation of the genetic material of the race. Treating the ill was only important if they could be fully restored for productivity in the Reich.

In a blatant example of forward-reversing, preventative medicine was used by doctors of the Third Reich to strengthen the "human genetic material" of those who were the strong of the Aryan race, while at the same time the same doctors weeded out the weak and exterminated them in order to preserve that same genetic material. As we in present-day America put more and more emphasis on making healthy people healthier, are we at the same time lowering our level of concern for those who are not, and can never be made, healthy? In the perspective of history, this is a question we cannot ignore.

Said one Auschwitz survivor appropriately: "The doctor . . . if not living in a moral situation . . . where limits are very clear . . . is very dangerous."[6] Unfortunately for the human race, that statement is still terrifying in its validity. When we see terms such as "quality of life" affecting what we believe about abortion, euthanasia, or refusal of treatment, just as the Nazi phrases "life unworthy of life" and "Final Solution" helped to justify medicalized killing to the German people, it should cause us alarm. When we hear about the need for racial purity, or read about any human being declared non-human, it should cause us alarm. For whenever it becomes acceptable to abuse the rights of anyone, it will inevitably become right to abuse the rights of others, including yours and mine. The enablement for such abuse will start with the distortion of words, which will then facilitate the behavior.

In clear biblical terms, the distortion and repetition of words which change our very beliefs are one way in which we can have our "conscience seared with a hot iron" (1 Timothy 4:2). For the Bible says that "in the latter times some shall depart from the faith, giving heed to seducing spirits, and doctrines of devils. Speaking lies in hypocrisy; having their conscience seared with a hot iron" (1 Timothy 4:1-2).

It is very possible that we in the free world may face times when, due to economic pressures, escalating medical costs, population explosion, food shortages, and even epidemics, individual life may become very cheap indeed. Euthanasia may not only be legalized, but it may become mandatory for various problems such as old age or chronic disease. Abortion, too, may become a decision for the state.

Yet to God who preserves our tears in a bottle (Psalm 56:8) and counts the very hairs on our head (Matthew 10:3), we will never cease to be precious as individuals. It is the love of God, above all else, which will hold us. If we are to survive in such times, and if we are to avoid being swept up by "seducing spirits" and the very "doctrines of devils," it is imperative that we remain true to our faith in the absolute authority of the Scriptures and in our commitment to the Lordship of Jesus Christ in our individual lives. For if Satan could do so he would deceive even the very elect (Mark 13:22).

While we cannot base either our theology or our ethics on love, if we truly love as the Scriptures command us we will be less tempted to tolerate evil simply because it does not *yet* touch us. In words spoken to his disciples prior to his crucifixion, Christ commanded them to "love one another, as I have loved you. Greater love hath no man than this, that a man lay down his life for his friends" (John 15:11-13).

At this time in man's history we in the free world are still called to love in small ways rather than in the more dramatic. With the exception of the abortion issue, it is not usual for us to be asked to save lives. Yet small acts of intolerance or prejudice, little compromises of truth and seemingly unimportant acts of selfishness can all be the seeds for future destruction. The major moral issues in this world which have so greatly influenced all of our lives in the last half century all started with small issues, tiny word changes, seemingly unimportant examples of forward-reversing.

Taking a Stand

I was born in Chicago at the outset of World War II. Before I can remember and before anyone in my Swedish family was aware of the atrocities which were going on "over there," the Jews were recognized in our family as God's chosen people.

My father had been looking for an apartment at a time when their availability was not great and his financial resources were small. At that time no one was required to rent to families with children, and so my sister and I were an added negative factor.

Finally he found the right one, he thought. The size and location were good for his family and his work. When he asked the price, the landlady, who was also Swedish, thought a moment and then quoted a price which was exorbitant. At first my father was angry and confused. Then as he thought the situation over quickly, he realized from some comments she had made earlier that the landlady thought he was Jewish. This was raw, blatant anti-Semitism!

Quietly he began to speak to her in his fluent Swedish. Relieved and pleased, the lady spoke back to him in Swedish and immediately the rent went down to half of the previous figure. To his eternal credit, my father turned to walk out of the apartment with the words, "No thank you. Nothing you could say and no rent reduction you could offer could make me live here now." It was a small incident. It was one man's private stand for righteousness. But as I was told the story when I was a child growing up, it made a lifelong impression on me, not only with regard to the Jews, but relating to the importance of one man's small stand against evil.

The Simon Wiesenthal Center in Los Angeles has a museum where articles belonging to Holocaust victims are displayed. Simple things are there, like wire eyeglasses, worn out shoes, hair taken from victims who died in the ovens, tattered pieces of clothing. My experience there was a moving one. I felt like I was in a place hallowed by the momentos of innocent suffering. I felt a strange need to fall to my knees in prayer.

Once again, too, I felt the need to help make sure such a holocaust never happens again. Never to the Jews. Never to those of us who claim the name of Christ. Never to anyone! And the only way to insure that a similar holocaust from a different direction aimed at perhaps a different group of people never occurs is for each of us to safeguard the rights of others as much as we safeguard our own. For if we don't stop error when it creeps into areas which affect other people, we will perhaps not be able to stop it when it enters an area which does affect us. We must indeed make a decision to love.

FIVE

"If I Should Die Before I Wake..."

A young healthy child well nursed is at a year old a most delicious, nourishing, and wholesome food, whether stewed, roasted, baked, or boiled, and I make no doubt that it will equally serve in a fricassee, or a ragout.[1]

When the satirist Jonathan Swift wrote these startling words in 1729, Ireland was in a crippled state economically. The country had just passed through a famine, and thousands had died of starvation. Swift wrote of using children for a food delicacy, not because he realistically thought this was a solution to Ireland's problems, but rather to shock people through his satire to some kind of compassion for women and children who were literally starving in the streets.

In an interesting aside, Swift added: "There is likewise another great advantage in my scheme, that it will prevent those voluntary abortions, and that horrid practice of women murdering their bastard children."[2]

For many today, as in Swift's time, it is not a good time to have a baby. For some women who wish to abort, the tragedy of rape or incest is involved. For others there can still be, even in our world, the disastrous consequences of a pregnancy which results from an impulsive act of sex outside of marriage. A marriage may be at stake, or a career.

Rejection by one's peers, while not as common for a child born out of wedlock as it was a few years ago, can still occur. For these women the choices which they must make can be as wrenching as they have ever been for all the women who have lived before them.

Even within a marriage, the prospect of having children is not always positive. A young woman sat in my counseling office and told me of the abortion which she had had a few months earlier. She had been married for two years, and then became pregnant. When she told her husband, his reaction was completely unexpected. "Get rid of it," he said roughly. "We can't afford a baby now. I'm not even sure I ever want one," he added. "If you don't get an abortion, our marriage is over."

After much arguing, the young woman decided to get the abortion because she didn't want to lose her husband. A few hours after the baby was aborted, the woman's husband sat down by her bed and said, "You know, honey, I've been thinking. Maybe we should go ahead and have a baby after all. Let's try and get pregnant again!"

Indeed, for many women today as in days past the frustration over an unwanted pregnancy and the pain over the idea of abortion is as acute as it has ever been. For these young women and for those who love them there are no easy answers. As one strong pro-life advocate said to me: "You know, I'm so adamantly against abortion, but if my seventeen-year-old daughter was raped, I don't know . . . I hope I'd have the courage."

Economic issues still exist too. Some women cannot afford to have another baby. For some, however, abortion has become simply a sloppy method of birth control which is neither fair to the unborn infant nor healthy for the mother. For a few women, abortion has degenerated into an act of total self-indulgence, where a woman terminates a pregnancy which will make her "fat for an upcoming cruise," or aborts one baby with the plan to conceive another within a few months when the new insurance will cover it or when it will simply be more convenient.

Abortion and Infanticide in the Bible

Abortion is not a new issue. In ancient societies, however, abortion was very risky for the mother, so the tendency was toward infanticide rather than abortion. For example, in the north African colony of Carthage during the fourth and third centuries B.C., at the time when the city had reached a peak in population, sociologists believe that ritual infanticide was used in order to control the population.

Says James Hoffmeier in his book *Abortion, A Christian Understanding and Response:*

> It was certainly safer to sacrifice a newborn than perform an abortion, and one could do it with the blessing of "the church and the state" in Canaan (and later in Carthage). For this reason, this author believes that the Old Testament is concerned with the practice of infant sacrifice, which might be considered the Canaanite counterpart to abortion. This may explain the silence of the Law and Prophets on abortion.[3]

In contrast to Carthage, ancient Egypt apparently did revere fetal life, since miscarried babies were mummified—showing that the Egyptian believed these infants would live in the next life:

> Two mummified stillborn babies were discovered in Tutankhamen's tomb, complete with miniature gold mummy cases. In a display case at the Field Museum of Natural History (Chicago), one can see a mummified fetus that was about four months old.[4]

Discussing further the Old Testament Law and child sacrifice, Hoffmeier states:

> The Law has much to say about child sacrifice; it is condemned in the strongest language. Leviticus 18:1-5 instructs Israel not to walk in the practices of the Canaanites, but after God's ordinances, and then specifies, "You shall not give any of your children to devote them by fire to Molech [or "as a sacrifice"] and

so profane the name of your God" (v. 21). According to Leviticus 20:2, the person who did this should be stoned to death. Deuteronomy 12:31 and 18:9-10 label the practice as *toebah*, "an abomination" to God. This means that child sacrifice is repugnant to God, completely the opposite of what he wanted.[5]

Furthermore,

The Hebrew language lacked a word for "fetus" or "embryo." The word *zera* means "seed," i.e., "semen" as well as "offspring." . . . This indicates that in Hebrew thought there was no distinction between a fetus and a baby.[6]

It would seem that if infanticide, the killing of a child, was repugnant to Jehovah God, then abortion, which was also considered to be the killing of a child, would be viewed as wrong. There are several Bible passages which show the value God places on life in the womb. Psalm 139:14-16 reads:

I am fearfully and wonderfully made: marvellous are thy works; and that my soul knoweth right well. My substance was not hid from thee, when I was made in secret, and curiously wrought in the lowest parts of the earth. Thine eyes did see my substance, yet being unperfect; and in thy book all my members were written, which in continuance were fashioned, when as yet there was none of them.

It is important to keep in mind that this description of the human body relates to the child who is yet in his mother's womb. Only in recent years, with some of our most modern technology, have we been able to see with our own eyes something of what the psalmist was talking about centuries ago.

Becoming more specific, according to Charles Spurgeon the psalmist's word "substance" could be translated as "life a ball yet to be unwound." He notes that such a translation was approved of by a number of scholars of his day,[7] while the clause "which in continuance were fashioned" is more accurately translated "my days were determined" before one of them was.[8] These translations not only validate God's concern with each living being prenatally, but they beautifully describe the genetic nature of this ball of life, which we call an embryo, in a way which outdoes any scientific knowledge of that time.

In a similar way, the prophet Jeremiah (1:5) describes the specific process by which God had made him:

Before I formed you in the womb I knew you intimately;
Before you were born I set you apart,
And appointed you a prophet to the nations.[9]

John Bright translates "knew you intimately" to mean "I chose you."[10] Andrew Blackwood elaborates the verse further by showing the series of acts of God involved in the formation of this great prophet *before* he ever entered this world: "I formed/I knew/I consecrated/I appointed."[11] Blackwood believes that the words translated "before you were born" would be better translated "before you came forth from the womb." Explains Blackwood: "The parallelism suggests the human situation in which God acts (*I formed you*) and man responds (*you came forth*)."[12] When God has implanted a life within the womb, it is an awesome thing indeed to tamper with that life and destroy it.

Something of God's viewpoint toward a person who would dare to destroy such a life is stated in Exodus 21:22-25. According to F. Delitzsch, accepted by many as the leading evangelical authority on the Hebrew Old Testament, this passage states that:

If men strove and thrust against a woman with child, who had come near or between them for the purpose of making peace, so that her children come out (come into the world), and no injury was done either to the woman or the child that was born, a pecuniary compensation was to be paid, such as the husband of the woman laid upon him, and he was to give it by (by an appeal to) arbitrators. A fine is imposed, because even if no injury had been done to the woman and the fruit of her womb, such a blow might have endangered life. But if injury occur (to the mother or the child), thou shalt give soul for soul, eye for eye, ... wound for wound: thus perfect retribution was to be made.[13]

This, in essence, is God's view of the sanctity of life of those both born and unborn.

Furthermore, the people of Israel had a very special incentive for protecting life in the womb. As Adam Clarke explains in commenting on this passage:

> As every man had some reason to think that the Messiah should spring from his family, therefore any injury done to a woman with child, by which the fruit of her womb might be destroyed, was considered a very heavy offence.[14]

Aborting the "Second Patient"

On January 22, 1973, the United States Supreme Court struck down the abortion laws of all fifty states, and, under certain conditions, legalized abortion-on-demand through the ninth month of pregnancy. Based on two related cases, Roe v. Wade and Doe v. Bolton, the Supreme Court (according to one writer's summary of the decisions) came to these conclusions:

> During the first three months of pregnancy, the state has no power to regulate abortion. The decision must be left entirely up to a woman and her physician.
>
> After the third month of pregnancy and until the fetus is viable (able to survive outside the mother's womb), the state can regulate abortion only to protect the health of the mother. Laws may be passed, for instance, requiring second-trimester abortions to be performed by a licensed physician or in a hospital setting.
>
> After a fetus has reached a point of viability, a state may regulate or even outlaw abortion, except when it is necessary "for the preservation of the life or health of the mother." If the life or health of the mother is threatened, any state laws regulating late-term abortions are overruled. The court then went on to

define "health" to include "all factors—physical, emotional, psychological, familial, and the woman's age—relevant to the well-being of the patient."[15]

The July 3, 1989, ruling of the Supreme Court relating to the Missouri law in Webster v. Reproductive Health Services made a start at returning the control of abortion to the states. But essentially Roe v. Wade still stands as the law at the time of the writing of this book.

It is more than ironic that after the high court declared this growing being in the womb to have no rights as a human being, the sixteenth edition of *Williams Obstetrics*, published in 1980, referred to the unborn child as the "second patient": "Happily we have entered an era in which the fetus can be rightfully considered and treated as our second patient."[16] *Williams Obstetrics* is a standard textbook in medical schools and is often referred to by practicing physicians.

Physicians are now routinely trained to treat this "second patient." They do diagnostic tests and perform surgery while the child is still in the womb. Furthermore, they take an oath before they become licensed doctors, an oath which would seem to include the unborn baby since that baby is, by their own definition, the "second patient." The Hippocratic Oath is the oldest of these oaths and the most well known, even though it is currently declining in popularity and usage. Still, to the public the Hippocratic Oath stands for those qualities and commitments which to us are most representative of the ideal physician. Included in that Oath are the words: "I will neither give a deadly drug to anybody if asked for it, nor will I make a suggestion to this effect. Similarly I will not give to a woman an abortive remedy. In purity and holiness I will guard my life and my art."[17]

Who is this "second patient" around whose life exists so much controversy? When the sperm and the egg first unite something called a zygote is produced. This one-celled individual with its complete set of forty-six chromosomes contains all the genetic material which make up a completely developed human being. At the moment of conception, the individual is unique and irreplaceable. This is a life, not a potential life, for at the point of conception there will never be another being just like it.

Within a few days this unique individual implants itself in the wall of the uterus and becomes known as the embryo. There it is nourished by the mother. But, wrapped in its own little sac, it is a totally unique and separate being from the mother. It is not a tumor, or an appendix. It is a separate being.

At eight weeks the baby is called a fetus. By this time it has a set of unique fingerprints which will never change. Whether or not this living being is considered a "baby" at this time seems to depend more upon what we want from the individual than upon any accuracy of definition. For example, a woman waiting for a gynecological examination in a clinic overheard the following conversation from the other side of the dividing curtain:

> "Your pregnancy test is positive," a nurse explained. "Do you want to keep the *fetus*?"
> After some added conversation which was not clearly audible, the patient apparently answered in the affirmative.
> "When would you like to come in to have the *baby* checked?" asked the nurse.

When the child's future was uncertain, it was a fetus. When it was a desired object of love, it became a baby. We abort fetuses. We care for babies. Terms like embryo and fetus—and even zygote—are handy technical terms which indicate the age of a baby. They were not invented in order to denote humanness or lack of it, and certainly not to determine whether or not the individual is worthy of life or death.

At what point does the fetus become a baby, if it is not truly human at the zygote or conception state? From a legal point of view, for those who do not consider conception to be the point at which human life begins, the word "viable" (the ability to live outside of the mother's womb) reverberates with unclarity and contradiction. State laws and court rulings have varied as to how old a fetus must be before it is "viable." Now that medical advances are very close to making it possible for the fetus to survive outside the mother's womb for the whole pregnancy—including conception in a petri dish—viability is becoming increasingly useless as a basis for when life begins.

In a 1983 decision, Supreme Court justice Sandra Day O'Connor pointed out two other problems with the viability standard:

> The Roe framework, then, is clearly on a collision course with itself. As the medical risks of various abortion procedures decrease, the point at which the State may regulate for reasons of maternal health is moved further forward to actual childbirth. As medical science becomes better able to provide for the separate existence of the fetus, the point of viability is moved further back toward conception.[18]

"Each of Them Babies"

To the common man, rather than the scientist or philosopher or lawyer, the question "what is life?" is sometimes quite simple. "Ron," one of the workmen who discovered the infamous container of 16,433 fetuses in a backyard in California, found one small body which had not been picked up when the container had spilled:

> The body lay sprawled in the soft earth. Ron squatted for another look. Four limbs were clearly distinguishable. At the end of two tiny arms, perfect fingers clenched into a fist. Five miniature toes crowned each little foot. There were even toenails. . . .
> Ron stared at the body fragments. . . .
> Ron guessed it was after three and school was out.
> Then, later that night, the dogs would come. . . .
> "I dug the heel of one boot into the dirt and scraped out a

mound of soft dirt. Then I rolled the tiny baby into the hole with my toe and covered it up. It was like a grave."[19]

Then Ron concluded with:

"I used to be religious, you know. But I'm not anymore. I'm just myself. But I believe in God. And I believe each of them babies was coming into this world with a job to do. This generation, our generation, can only go so far. Then the next one has to take over. That's the way I learned it. But a big part of the next generation is mangled up and thrown away like garbage. Discarded like them babies in the container."[20]

I hope Ron has discovered Psalm 139:13-16, this time quoted from *The Living Bible* paraphrase:

You made all the delicate, inner parts of my body, and knit them together in my mother's womb. Thank you for making me so wonderfully complex! It is amazing to think about. Your workmanship is marvelous—and how well I know it. You were there while I was being formed in utter seclusion! You saw me before I was born and scheduled each day of my life before I began to breathe. Every day was recorded in your Book!

It seems that God himself was saying with Ron: "Each of them babies was coming into this world with a job to do."

Methods of Abortion

Apart from the moral issues of viability, the longer the pregnancy the more complicated the abortion procedure and the greater the physical pain to both mother and child.

In the early stages of pregnancy intrauterine devices and the progestogen-only pill ("mini-pill") can be used to prevent the zygote from implanting itself in the uterine wall. Other methods of abortion in the first trimester are:

Suction curettage: Under a local anaesthetic a suction tube is inserted into the mouth of the womb. The amniotic membrane and fluid are removed first; and then the baby is suctioned away, piece by piece, with the head removed last. Next the placenta is removed, if possible, from the wall of the uterus. Then the uterine wall is scraped in order to remove any remaining tissue of the embryo.

Dilatation and curettage (D & C): In this procedure the uterus is scraped first and then suctioned.

After the first trimester, a frequently used method involves injecting a substance into the amniotic sac which will kill the fetus and cause the mother to deliver a dead baby. Saline is perhaps the most commonly used substance. The child breathes and swallows the solution and is literally burned. In a saline abortion the baby takes an hour or more to die. There is also the very real possibility of a live delivery with a damaged baby.

The use of prostaglandins, hormones which can be used to cause violent contractions resulting in the expulsion of the fetus, is another method of chemical abortion. This procedure can be painful for the mother and can once again, with even greater predictability than with saline solution, result in the birth of a live baby. The possibility of a live birth is so great with the use of prostaglandins that the pharmaceutical company which makes them lists live births as a possible complication! There are also unpleasant systemic side affects for the mother, such as nausea and cramping.

A frequently used method of abortion after the first trimester is dilatation and evacuation (D & E). Forceps are inserted which are used to cut the fetus into pieces, or the physician may have to manually pull apart the baby in order to pull it out, again, piece by piece. That largest piece of the child, the head, must be crushed with the use of forceps and removed. It then becomes essential to reassemble the pieces of the infant once it has been aborted, in order to make sure that no pieces have been left inside the mother.

It is aspects of abortion technique like reassembling the pieces, the sound of breaking bones as the baby is removed, and just the experience of watching the baby on an ultrasound before killing it that have made many physicians as well as nurses and technicians resign from participation in abortion procedures. After losing his daughter when she was hit by a car in front of his own house, one physician chose to stop doing abortions. "If you lose a child, you look at things differently," he said. "What was once uncomfortable becomes intolerable. You feel that you're destroying a human being for money, like a paid assassin."[21]

If the baby is not aborted until very late in the pregnancy, one of the techniques that may be used is a hysterotomy. The hysterotomy is a surgical procedure like the caesarean section, differing in that it seeks to terminate the life of the baby rather than save it. Once again, what frequently results is a live baby and considerable risk for the mother. Sometimes the umbilical cord is tied in order to kill the baby if it is still alive. At times babies have been left on counters to see if they make it on their own, unobserved and uncared for, with the result that many do not. However, the live, approximately two-pound babies that can result from a hysterotomy are a source of great embarrassment and perplexity to the abortionist, so this technique is increasingly avoided.

It is an irony of abortion that it forces a physician to forward-reverse from healer to executioner. And for many it has become a business. One physician in New York said with honesty: "It's highly profitable. I could do three abortions in my office in an hour and a half, and make more than caring for a woman nine months and delivering a baby."[22] In order to achieve this "businesslike" viewpoint, a lot of mental games are played. The baby is called everything from "fetus" to a "product of conception." Just as Hitler called the killing of Jews the "final solution" so the abortionist calls the killing of babies the "termination of a pregnancy." The muted, meaningless terms serve as enablements, keeping the physician from facing what he or she is really doing. The physician who aborts babies forward-reverses from healing to killing by viewing the whole process as one continuum: treating his patient, the mother. Sometimes as a further enablement the mother is called the "potential mother," and the term "second patient" is completely blocked from the doctor's mind. The "product of conception" is only treated as the "second patient" if it is to be kept, in which case, to at least the mother, it becomes "my baby."

Do the Unborn Feel Pain?

There has been considerable debate over whether or not the unborn child can feel pain. In a speech on January 30, 1986, to the National Religious Broadcasters Convention, President Reagan contended that fetuses do indeed suffer "long and agonizing" pain. This statement, though contradicted by some, made an impact on many of us who up to that time may not have considered to any real degree the issue of fetal pain. A letter to Reagan from Dr. Richard Schmidt and Dr. Fred Hofmeister, both past presidents of the American College of Obstetricians and Gynecologists, supported his position.

According to James Hoffmeier, "Anesthesiologist Vincent Collins, a professor at the University of Illinois Medical Center, says that nervous-system structures are in place six to eight weeks after conception and can respond to painful stimuli. . . ." Hoffmeier continues:

> In a conversation with me, Dr. Richard Schmidt indicated "that those who defend abortion often confuse or ignore the distinction between feeling pain and forming an idea of pain. Most of us have at some time or other experienced a sudden, severe pain, reacted vigorously to it by withdrawing, jumping or crying out—these reactions occurring a perceptible moment before our higher cortical centers have identified the specific nature or relative severity of the pain or even its exact location. Is it intense heat or cold, or cutting or crushing? Is it one toe or the entire foot? It is only this integrating function which is incompletely developed in the fetus at a stage when it can clearly be demonstrated to perceive ("feel") and react purposefully to a painful stimulus.[23]

Periodically we see on the evening news a story where a newborn baby has been pulled out of a trash container. Usually the child is lovingly cared for and the abandoning parent is searched for with great indignation. One such incident was shown on the news this morning. A public health worker stated with emotion that, had the baby not cried out when he did and thereby been discovered by a passerby, he might have died. Truly we are confused! Twenty-four hours before he was dumped in the trash, the baby could have been aborted. He would have been considered by these same public health officials to be a "fetus," not human, a "product of conception." As a victim of hysterotomy he might have been left to die in a pail of water. Or if the pregnancy of which he was a product had been terminated with the use of saline solution, he would have been burned to death. Instead, by being born, he merely changed his address from the danger of the womb to the safety of planet earth, and, if he could reason at this age, even he would have been surprised at his change in treatment. He would have thanked his frightened mother for dumping him in the trash, where he could be rescued and lovingly cared for and adopted, instead of killing him in his previous residence, the womb. In this case the trash barrel was safer than the womb!

By the use of conflicting terminology and by refusing to see the illogic of what we are doing, abortion has continued for a long time in a society which has more would-be adoptive parents than adoptable babies, and in a scientific atmosphere which invests inordinate amounts of time and money on fertility, alternate reproductive techniques and surgical procedures for the unborn fetus. Yet at the time of the writing of this book, a baby is aborted once every twenty seconds.

We have taken the clause, "If I should die before I wake," out of our children's bedtime prayer because it is considered too traumatic a thought, and yet many children watch unspeakable violence on television in their own living rooms. Furthermore, many children are aware that their brothers and sisters have died in the womb before they ever had a chance to wake into life on this earth. For children are often very aware of the death, even the death in the womb, of a sibling. As one little girl said to me of the miscarriage her mother had in the first trimester: "The baby died, but God took her and she's in heaven now." Fortunately for this little girl's mental health later on in life, the baby who died had been genuinely wanted. There will be no traumatic revelations later on.

We are a society which has made great efforts to prevent child abuse. In some countries, like Sweden, spanking has even been abolished; and yet in both Sweden and the United States, laws protecting children have been enacted right alongside those laws which have abolished the rights of the unborn. We can kill babies, but we can't beat them.

In the still remarkable book, *Whatever Happened to the Human Race?* by Francis Schaeffer and C. Everett Koop, M.D., the authors state with blunt logic:

> Is it not logical, after all, that if one can legally kill a child a few months before birth, one should not feel too bad about roughing him up a bit (without killing him) after he is born? Parents who are apprehended for child abuse must feel that the system is somewhat unfair in that they can be arrested for beating their child, whereas people who kill their infant before birth (at an "earlier age") go scot-free—in fact have society's approval.[24]

And if killing seems like too harsh a word, let us look at abortion once again with cold reason. Something in that womb moves, sucks its thumb, eats, eliminates, and grows. Many studies even show that by the time a child is born he or she recognizes his mother's voice; and there is every evidence that the unborn child is influenced by the music which the mother listens to during her pregnancy. Then that something is attacked in the womb and ceases to be. Regardless of whether or not abortion is legal, certainly one can most appropriately say that, in an abortion, the organism in the womb dies. It no longer exists as a living being, and like any dead thing it rots and disintegrates. Just as it once resembled life, it now resembles death. It has been killed.

It is argued that the issue here is a woman's right over her own body. Yet we do not give a woman, or a man, the right to kill her own body, or the right to abuse that body with drugs. She can't sell her body for prostitution. Furthermore, supposing for the sake of argument that in some contradictory way this unborn child does not possess individual rights, what right then does a woman have to claim that it belongs only to her? Isn't this being the result of the union of the egg *and* the sperm? What happens to the rights of the father? Yet, regardless of anyone else's rights, if an unborn baby infringes upon the rights of a woman's comfort or freedom or privacy, some would argue that the baby can be killed.

A Crime Against Humanity;
A Crime Against Nature

After World War II when war criminals were tried at Nuremberg, a new charge was raised in international law: the charge of crimes against humanity. Up to this time the kind of atrocities which had been committed during this war had not been thought of in international law. When charged with crimes against humanity:

> No defendant could claim the protection of having obeyed orders from a superior, though superior orders might be considered by the Tribunal as a mitigating factor in sentencing. The denial of the defense of superior orders has often been called the "Nuremberg Principle."[25]

Those of us who are citizens of those countries of the Allied forces which defeated the Third Reich have been very harsh in our judgment of the German people who "did nothing" to prevent some of the atrocities which were committed by Hitler's armies. The declaration of non-humanness regarding the Jews, the handicapped, the blacks, the gypsies: this designation enabled not only the killing but the experimenting which was conducted in the concentration camps of Hitler's Third Reich. It was in the thinking of the German people and in the laws which were enacted as a result of that thinking where debate and protest needed to start. Once the killing machines were started up it became very difficult to stop them.

As the law of the land in the United States shows signs of fluctuating and as we debate when a baby is a human being, it might be well for us to consider the atrocities of the Third Reich and ask ourselves whether or not we are committing our own atrocities by the same enablement which was used by the Nazis: "Non-human." Non-humanness permits the tolerance of atrocities. To decide that someone is non-human and can therefore be torn apart, or burned, and killed, is to assume awesome responsibility indeed. Moreover, just because something is legal, does not automatically make it either moral or humane. Our involvement in World War II should have taught us that.

Abortion could be considered a crime against humanity; it is a crime against *nature* as well. It is natural for a woman to protect the life of her young. In the Book of Job in the Old Testament we learn that some living creatures do not have this basic human instinct:

> The ostrich flaps her wings grandly, but has no true motherly love. She lays her eggs on top of the earth, to warm them in the dust. She forgets that someone may step on them and crush them, or the wild animals destroy them. She ignores her young as though they weren't her own, and is unconcerned though they die, for God has deprived her of wisdom (Job 39:13-17, TLB).

At a time when they had greatly sinned and were enduring God's wrath, God compares his own people with the ostrich:

> Even the jackals feed their young, but not my people, Israel. They are like cruel desert ostriches, heedless of their babies'

cries. The children's tongues stick to the roofs of their mouths for thirst, for there is not a drop of water left. Babies cry for bread but no one can give them any.... Tender-hearted women have cooked and eaten their own children; thus they survived the siege (Lamentations 4:3-4, 10, TLB).

God's people were in the worst of circumstances. Famine and death were all around them. This, like Ireland during the days of Jonathan Swift, was not an easy time to have a child. Yet God seems to condemn their behavior in spite of the difficulty of the times. It would also seem that God's wrath is against these women, not only for the neglect and mistreatment of their *born* children, but also the abuse of their unborn. For the comparison is made between their mistreatment of children and the ostrich's mistreatment of its born as well as unborn young. Once again the Bible makes no distinction between the born and the unborn. They are both children. What seems to matter to God is the presence or lack of instinctive maternal love.

In Isaiah 66:13 God compares his own care of those he loves with that of the normal attitude of a mother toward her infant, and by so doing God emphasizes his own view of natural maternal love. He says: "As one whom his mother comforteth, so will I comfort you." Such love comforts and protects with its very life. It does not kill. It is tender, not cruel. Such love would fulfill perhaps more than any other human love the high standard in the New Testament of that love which lays down its very life.

"There Are Other Alternatives"

A woman in her early thirties came into my office with a small child, who obediently played with the toys while her mother and I talked. Susan looked deceptively composed. She was dressed with style, as was her little girl, and she seemed proud of her husband's job as an accountant.

Then her story came out. "I've been having an affair for

a year," she said. "I've been very careful, and no one knows anything about it. But now I'm pregnant, quite obviously with his child since I haven't made love to my husband in at least four months. I can't believe that I am actually going to have an abortion, but I have no choice. I have an appointment for tomorrow."

"There are other alternatives," I found myself saying. I explained to her, as I do to anyone consulting me about abortion, that while I am personally opposed to abortion I was willing to help her sort through the various alternatives and her own conflicting feelings without rejecting her if she ultimately disagreed with me. It is my responsibility as a counselor to provide an atmosphere where such matters can be discussed freely and to accept someone's conclusions whether or not they agree with mine. But it is also my right as a human being, and my obligation, to state what my position is. Most people can handle my disagreement if that disagreement is stated in love.

"There are other alternatives!" Even I paused as I said the words. What could any woman conceivably do, in this kind of situation, without hurting many innocent people? Yet she grabbed at my words like someone gulping down cool water in a parched desert. She left my office with greater peace about her situation than even I felt.

She kept the medical appointment, but decided against the abortion. I didn't see her again until after the baby was born. She brought him in to see me when he was about three months old. Under these circumstances, keeping the baby rather than putting him up for adoption would not have worked for many people; but in Susan's case her husband was able to love the child for himself rather than hate him for his paternity. The biological father relinquished his rights, and Susan's husband adopted the child. God had been kind and given her joy out of sorrow, hope out of hopelessness. He had rewarded her desire to obey him in spite of all the horrible potential, humanly speaking. He had healed where no healing seemed possible.

Most young women are not lacking in maternal instincts. Most physicians would rather heal than kill. Sometimes we need to hear words as simple as, "there are other alternatives."

For those of us who oppose abortion, it is essential that we oppose in love, or all of our good deeds are nothing. Somewhere a long while back I heard a story of a woman who had witnessed the trial of Nazi leader Adolph Eichmann in Israel. Eichmann's commitment to the eradication of the Jewish people from the face of the earth was unquenchable. As the woman watched Eichmann's face and witnessed the hate written across it, she recalled that she had seen that hate somewhere before. Then with a start she realized that the only other place she had ever seen that extreme of hate had been on the face of one of those who had witnessed against Eichmann. The victimizer and the victim had become united in their hate!

In the area of abortion it is possible to so condemn a frightened and desperate woman or even, in some cases, an ambivalent doctor, to the point that our hate becomes worse than the deed which we condemn. "If I were burned alive for preaching the gospel but didn't love others, it would be of no value whatever" (1 Corinthians 13:3, TLB). "If you love someone you will be loyal to him no matter what the cost. You will always believe in him, always expect the best of him, and always stand your ground in defending him" (1 Corinthians 13:7, TLB).

Loving people when we disagree with them is very difficult for most of us. If we aren't careful we may find that nothing can be more harsh than righteous disagreement. Love, on the other hand, does not imply that we change our minds about what we believe. It means we love in spite of the conflict in belief. Such love is not predicated upon the change in belief of the other person. But such love does, at times, enable the other person to re-think his or her position. Love is a powerful force for change. Hate seldom causes people to change. Indeed, it can prevent positive growth.

For those who have killed the unborn and repent, God still says to them as he said to Jerusalem :

> Then will I sprinkle clean water upon you, and ye shall be clean. ... A new heart also will I give you, and a new spirit will I put within you: and I will take away the stony heart out of your flesh, and I will give you a heart of flesh ... and ye shall be my people, and I will be your God (Ezekiel 36:25-28).

SIX

Opening Pandora's Box

A child's version of the ancient myth of Pandora's box reads in part:

> Pandora was perfect—almost! The gods had given her beauty, charm, and gracefulness. But along with these great gifts, Pandora was given curiosity. Not just a little curiosity. But enough curiosity so that she had to know everything about everything.
>
> Before Pandora went to live in the world of people, the king of the gods gave her a box and told her never to open it. Never!
>
> Pandora tried to obey. She stared at the box. She touched it with cool slender fingers. She tried locking it away in a cupboard. But her curiosity was too great.
>
> "Just a peek!" she thought. "Just one peek."
>
> She opened the box . . .
>
> That one peek was one peek too many. Out popped all the bad things of the world—greed, envy, gossip, meanness . . . and on and on.[1]

In a February 1975 decision West Germany's Supreme Court banned abortion-on-demand during the first trimester of pregnancy, stating that:

> "We cannot ignore the educational impact of abortion on the respect for life." The German court reasoned that if abortion were made legal for any and every reason during the first

trimester, it would prove difficult to persuade people that second-and-third-trimester fetuses deserve protection simply because they are a few weeks older. The court apparently feared that what would happen to older fetuses could also happen to children after birth.[2]

In the United States the 1973 Roe v. Wade decision resulted in what the high court in West Germany had essentially feared: it opened up the way for medicalized killing in this country. Doctors could kill, and indeed might be obligated to do so. The fact that in the first ten years following this decision over ten million babies were killed is tragic. Yet even more tragic is that, regardless of the present legal status of abortion and in spite of the legal fluctuations which may continue regarding abortion, the fact that as a nation we could ever legally kill each other has opened up a Pandora's box of medicalized killing which will be difficult to close up again. We have found that it is not so hard to kill after all!

Mystery writer Agatha Christie reiterates in her mystery books that it is the first murder which is the most difficult. After that it is easy to kill:

A useful term in this connection is primicide, the first murder. When it is first suggested that we do a murderous deed, we may respond, "But that would be murder!" After we have done it once, or maybe twice, that response loses some of its force of conviction. As a barrier to evil, novelty is a one-time thing; it cannot be reinstated. In the 1930s a hit man for Murder, Inc. was on trial. The prosecutor asked him how he felt when committing a murder. He in turn asked the prosecutor how he felt when he tried his first case in court, to which the prosecutor allowed that he was nervous, but he got used to it. "It's the same with murder," observed the hit man, "you get used to it."[3]

This nation has agonized more over the abortion issue than any other social issue of our time. But once we opened the box, so to speak, which allowed the killing of the unborn, we did as the German court predicted: we made it easier to kill babies in any trimester. From that point it has been easy to think about killing the newborn, or the old, or the sick or the depressed—or anyone whom we feel has poor quality of life—life unworthy of life.

Abortion itself has become easier as time has gone by. As I observed in chapter 4, it used to be that when pregnant girls would talk to me regarding the pros and cons of having an abortion, the conversation usually revolved around the issue of whether or not this unborn fetus was a human being. "When does human life start?" was the issue. Gradually those discussions became unimportant, as many young girls seemed more blatantly willing to kill what they now viewed as an unborn baby. As one girl stated with no prompting from me. "I know that it's not fair to the baby and I know that the baby is a human being, but I don't want to ruin my senior year in high school. Also, I find it harder to think of giving the baby up for adoption once I have it than I do of aborting it now." Killing has become easy.

The Right of Choice for *Her* Own Body

A major justification which I hear for abortion, from those who really don't like the idea of killing babies, is that, if these babies are born and then raised by their natural mother, they will not have a chance for a good life. I find it hard, however, to justify killing for such a reason! Where do we stop with that kind of logic? Do we kill children who are wards of the court? Do we kill all juvenile delinquents? Do we kill victims of child abuse so they will no longer be victims? Actually the logic becomes ridiculous. You can't protect someone by killing them. Also, there is in each human being, regardless of his or her circumstances, the glorious opportunity for choice. He may be fated to the circumstances of his birth, but he is not fated to the course of his whole life.

An elderly woman named Ida asked me about this book as I was writing it. "What is your view on abortion?" she asked. Then as I started a lengthy answer, she interrupted with, "Are you for or against it?"

"Against." I answered simply.

"Oh no!" she replied, almost in horror as she drew back. "I just think of all those children out there who are beaten and starved, who would have been better off if they had been aborted."

Then she went into a lengthy story of her own childhood. She and her three sisters had been given to an orphanage when her mother couldn't afford to keep them. As a child her hands had been placed in boiling water as a punishment and food was forcibly shoved down her little sister's throat when she didn't want to eat. One sister, as a punishment, was put into a dark closet where she became hysterical when spiders crawled over her in the dark. One was molested by a doctor when she was sick. In general, their treatment by those who should have cared was appalling and abusive.

In the course of her life, Ida had tried to kill herself several times. Even as we talked, she expressed the wish that she could have been aborted from the womb.

Fortunately I knew something of her life in the recent past. She had cared for several sick ladies. She had faithfully visited a bedridden child who was a ward of the state. Once, while walking by a homeless lady on a windy corner, she had taken off her own coat and given it to her.

I reminded her of some of these acts of kindness, and with genuineness of feeling Ida expressed how happy it had made her to be of help to people who were in need. "Indeed," she replied, "these past few years, when I've had more time to just help people, have been the happiest years of my life."

I continued: "There are a lot of people who wouldn't have been helped if you had been aborted, Ida. The lady freezing on the corner would have gone on freezing. The sick ladies who needed care might not have had anyone to help them. And you and I both know that no one else was remotely interested in visiting that sick child. Even her own parents had abandoned her."

There was a silence. Then I asked my question: "When

you think about these people you have helped, do you still believe in abortion? Do you still believe there are throw-away kids? Do you still wish you had been aborted?"

In a voice more gentle than I had ever heard from her before, she replied: "No, I'll never say that again. I just never thought of it that way before."

I was glad that I had asked the question, and glad for her answer. I was glad she had been given the chance to evaluate her own life rather than having had someone else do it for her before she was even born. I was glad that *she* had been given the right of choice for *her* own body.

Brave New Experimentation

The Pandora's box of abortion has also made it morally easier to experiment in the area of alternative reproduction techniques. Indeed we have a schizophrenic conflict as doctors seek to compete with God in the creation of life while at the same time exhibiting a blatant disregard for human life in terms of abortion and euthanasia. The frenzied quest for exploring newer horizons of medical experimentation, coupled with a desire for children (which often seems to focus on fulfilling the needs of the adult rather than on giving life to the baby for its own sake), have made such a conflict possible.

For example, in the procedure called in vitro fertilization, conception occurs in a petri dish. Because the procedure is costly and involved, several embryos are desirable. More than one of these embryos are then implanted in the woman's womb with the hope that at least one will attach itself to the uterine wall and survive. Depending on the technology available, the remaining embryos can be thrown down a drain, frozen and implanted at a future date, adopted out, used for fetal experimentation, or they can be "farmed" in order to provide tissue or organs for transplant purposes.[4]

Most of these uses for the embryos are contingent upon

viewing them as something less than human, as potential life rather than as a human being. The notion that the life of these embryos is less than human enables the decision to kill that life; and the right to kill a human embryo enables a freedom to deal with that embryo as one wishes. No laws can then protect its rights as a human being.

To want children is a God-given desire. But that desire must always be subordinated to the will of God. It can never be right, for example, to kill embryos in order to have a baby in the process. The end still does not justify the means.

There are certainly aspects of alternate reproductive techniques which can appropriately be used to help couples have children without infringing upon the rights of the unborn and without violating basic morality. For some women an example is in the area of artificial insemination. While with in vitro fertilization conception occurs outside of the body, with artificial insemination the sperm is artificially introduced into the body, usually with the help of a physician. If the sperm is a donor sperm some may feel that, while the act is not one of adultery, the actual conception may be considered an adulterous one.

However, artificial insemination is often used simply to enhance the effectiveness of the husband's sperm by concentrating the specimen down and injecting it directly into the uterus. Some would feel that even this kind of artificial insemination is wrong because medical technology helps along the process of conception. Yet in some ways that is no more logical than saying that if you have pneumonia you shouldn't take penicillin because it stops the natural process of dying from pneumonia! We already accept medical intervention by medication and surgery. The big question for most of us is not whether any of this modern technology is right; the question is how much of it is right.

Some, particularly in the Roman Catholic Church, have raised the question of whether conception apart from intercourse can be right, even where the egg and the sperm belong to the couple involved and where there is no discarding or abuse of unused embryos.

In the Vatican view, couples must combine the "unitive" (sexual) and the "procreative" aspects of marriage. Artificial methods of producing children consider only procreation, says Rome, while artificial methods of birth control consider only the sexual aspect. Since artificial insemination and in vitro fertilization bypass the normal "conjugal act," neither method is allowed.[5]

Even those who don't totally adhere to the Roman Catholic point of view should not disregard the problems surrounding the issue of conception apart from intercourse. Of the couples I have seen who are using a combination of available fertility methods, even those as simple as fertility medication combined with the careful timing of intercourse, many develop marital problems because the sex act becomes mechanistic and timed. Love-making is no longer focused upon the expression of love but on the goal of impregnation. When this happens it is sad to watch a couple who once had a good marriage introduce a child into a home where there no longer is a bond of love between the parents. The child becomes focused on in a possessive way rather than being loved unselfishly, and often he or she eventually becomes the object of a custody fight in a divorce proceeding.

In speaking of the variety of alternate reproductive techniques which are being developed, and their result on marriage and the family, biologist Leon Kass states succinctly:

> What is new is nothing more radical than the divorce of the generation of new human life from human sexuality, and ultimately, from the confines of the human body, a separation which began with artificial insemination and which will finish with ectogenesis, the full laboratory growth of a baby from sperm to term.[6]

On a more philosophical level Kass continues:

> Is there possibly some wisdom in the mystery of nature that joins the pleasure of sex, the inarticulate longing for union, the communication of love, and the deep and partly articulate desire for children in the very activity by which we continue the chain of human existence? Is biological parenthood a built-in

"device" elected to promote the adequate caring for posterity?
Before we embark on new modes of reproduction we should
consider the meaning of the union of sex, love, and procreation,
and the meaning and consequences of its cleavage. . . .

I am arguing that the laboratory production of human
beings is no longer *human* procreation, that making babies in
laboratories—even perfect "babies"—means a degradation of
parenthood.[7]

Christians often cling to absolutes, to answers which are
"black and white." "Greys" bother us. Yet as Christians we
are a priesthood of believers (1 Peter 2:5), with an indwelling
Holy Spirit who, we are told, will lead us into all truth (John
14:15-17, TLB). Surely this includes helping us discern God's
will in these grey areas.

Rarely has that leading been so needed as in dealing with
the current issues of medical ethics. In the area of alternative
reproductive techniques, right and wrong are not always
clear. Many women who come into my counseling office
have difficulty discerning the will of God for them in these
areas. As one woman said: "I want God's will above all else,
and if God doesn't want me to have a baby I must be willing
for that. But if some of these techniques can be used of God
to help me get pregnant, then I want to use them." To those
of us who counsel such women, or who are their family or
friends, this is an arena in which to exercise the love of God.
I doubt that anyone reading this book will agree on every
issue. Many will disagree on many issues. But the challenge
of our time as Christians is to act in love toward those who
disagree with us without compromising our own beliefs. For
while we cannot base our ethics on "what is most loving," we
can act out those beliefs in love.

The Return of Eugenics

Research in alternate reproductive methods is not the only area which has been affected by this opening of Pandora's box to medicalized killing. The whole area of eugenics is being talked about again after some thirty years of unpopularity following the fall of the Third Reich. Eugenics relates to the development of techniques aimed at perfecting the human species. Hitler's brand of eugenics involved the concept of scientific racism, where so-called impurities were removed from the human race, and, in his case, the Aryan race was promoted.

Many practices which violate the sanctity of life can arise out of this renewed interest in eugenics. For example, many fear that using fetal tissue in experimentation or even in the direct treatment of disease will eventuate into the commercialization of fetuses, where the unborn are bought and sold to the highest bidder. Ironically, the rights of women could be violated also . . . when women become simply breeders. Such a possibility is not just out there in the "twilight zone"; already families have proposed the idea of conceiving a child and then aborting it for the experimental treatment of another family member.[8] In a country where medical technology has out-priced the average pocketbook, it is conceivable that women may someday breed their own offspring for economic returns, or in exchange for medical treatment for a loved one.

Nor are the newborn safe any more. In order to use newborn organs and/or tissues for transplantation into those with diseases like diabetes or Parkinson's, it has become necessary for some to try to admit to a new morality where it is right to kill the defective newborn or to re-define death so that those infants born with most of their brain missing (anencephalic) would be declared dead.[9]

Many of the most respected scientists of our day favor the right to kill defective newborns. In May 1973, four months after the passage of Roe v. Wade, Nobel Prize-winning scientist Dr. James Watson said that:

If a child was not declared alive until three days after birth, then all parents could be allowed the choice that only a few are given under the present system [that is, to have their defective offspring killed]. The doctor could allow the child to die if the parents so chose and save a lot of misery and suffering.[10]

In 1978 another Nobel prize winner, Dr. Francis Crick, gave his opinion that "no newborn infant should be declared human until it has passed certain tests regarding its genetic endowment . . . if it fails these tests it forfeits the right to live."[11]

Once again the views of Joseph Fletcher come into view to help us make the transition, this time to the nursery and then to the general population. From Fletcher's viewpoint, "It is reasonable to describe infanticide as a post-natal abortion."[12]

Furthermore, as Fletcher says elsewhere:

If we are morally obliged to put an end to a pregnancy when an amniocentesis reveals a terribly defective fetus, we are equally obliged to put an end to a [cancer] patient's hopeless misery when a brain scan reveals advanced brain metastases.[13]

And so the process of medicalized killing proceeds in a hundred different directions, with each step enabled by the previous step. If the Nazis simply went too far, as many now say in their own defense of the present renewal of interest in eugenics, some of us would feel that we too have already gone too far.

Infanticide is practiced today (see *Death in the Nursery*, and *Fighting for Life*, cited in the bibliography), but its practice is cloaked in euphemisms and a conspiracy of silence. In the words of C. Everett Koop:

Semantics have made infanticide palatable by never referring to the practice by that word, but by using such euphemisms as "selection." "Starving a child to death" becomes "allowing him to die." Although infanticide is not talked about even in professional circles, the euphemisms are. It is all illegal, but the law has turned its back. The day will come when the argument will be as it was for abortion: "Let's legalize what is already happening." Then what is legal is right. Attention will then be turned to the next class of individuals that might be exterminated without too loud an outcry.[14]

The end result of medicalized killing is the use of the medical profession to kill those whom society at any given time deems unworthy to live. What starts as mercy killing will turn into decisions made for people by those who don't want to care for them or by those who want their organs or by those who simply think they know the right definition of *quality of life*.

Willful Self-deception

Using doctors to kill lends a sense of respectability to the whole process. Hitler, too, insisted that the killing be medicalized. But what then prevents the patient from questioning the motives of his own doctor's treatment? What prevents him from asking whether his physician is approaching him as a healer or as an executioner? What makes the patient so sure that something about himself may not have placed him on the next-to-be-killed list?

A physician who survived the death camps, Dr. Ella Lingens-Reiner, pointed to the distant chimneys and asked Nazi doctor Fritz Klein:

> "How can you reconcile that with your [Hippocratic] oath as a doctor?" His answer was, "Of course I am a doctor and I want to preserve life. And out of respect for human life, I would remove a gangrenous appendix from a diseased body. The Jew is the gangrenous appendix in the body of mankind."[15]

Human nature has great powers of self-deception which are being put to remarkable use in the area of medicalized killing.

In 1949 Dr. Leo Alexander, U.S. consultant to the Nuremberg trials wrote: "It is the first seemingly innocent step away from principle that frequently decides a career of crime. Corrosion begins in microscopic proportions."[16] In recent history we have watched good nations like Germany escalate killing until a whole race was almost exterminated just because they belonged to a certain race. The Jews were not defective, or unborn, or retarded, or terminally ill. They were Jews. And that was all they had to be to become the focus of Hitler's extermination plan. Today it is abortion; tomorrow it is infanticide; the next day it will be voluntary euthanasia. And then it will become forced euthanasia.

What a tolerance of medicalized killing does to a people who permit it is perhaps more frightening then even the killing itself. When life is so valuable to me that I have to kill others to be able to afford my own life, or use dead babies in order to preserve my own existence, then I have indeed cheapened the value of my own life. What a far cry such an attitude is from the ideal of giving one's life to save the lives of others, as exemplified by those who have died on the battlefields of our nation's history. The ideal of giving one's life for another has kept us a nation worthy of our respect. But how will we be able to respect a nation of people who willingly sacrifice the lives of others so that they themselves might live?

President Bush declared in his 1989 Inaugural Address that a man cannot judge his worth by possessions alone, reminding us to beware of a crass selfishness which reduces the worth of a man rather than enhancing it. Yet because we are human, for most of us the dangers we face in the issues relating to medicalized killing will be realized most effectively only when we face how these dangers could affect us specifically.

A contemporary paraphrase of the words of Pastor Niemöller might read:

They came for the unborn, but I wasn't unborn—so I walked away.

They came for the newborn and took their organs, but I was not newborn—so I chose not to know.

They came for the very old, but I wasn't old yet—so I said nothing.

They came for the incurably ill and those suffering from what they called "poor quality of life"; but I liked my quality of life—so I did nothing.

But then they came for me, and I didn't even know why—and there was no one left to do anything.

All of this discussion on the opening of Pandora's box and medicalized killing may be difficult to read and unpleasant to think about, but it will become desperately important to each of us when it suddenly relates to *me*. What will I do when my baby *must* be aborted because no defectives are allowed? Will I find myself in a back alley having that baby in secrecy, to say nothing of raising it in hiding? What will I do when, as happened in Germany, my physically fit son comes back from fighting for his country and is put to death because he is now handicapped? What will I do when I am old and cannot afford outside help and am therefore put to death? My "right to die" will have become my obligation to die. My so-called rights will have turned to curse me.

SEVEN

Touching
the Face of Evil

An elderly couple sat down by their friends in a restaurant. The man turned to one friend and said: "When my time comes, just give me an overdose. . . . I don't want to be a burden to my children."

The friend later related the incident to me and commented: "Our friends are the most wonderful people. They are so thoughtful. If everyone were like those people you wouldn't have to write *Life on the Line*."

"You're wrong," I replied. "They *are* who I'm writing this book for . . . the nice people of this world! People who not only feel right about calling the shots on their own life and death, but actually feel noble and responsible in so doing. The nice people in the world *enable* the not-so-nice people. They are the ones who often set the precedent for the acceptance of, not just voluntary euthanasia or so-called 'mercy killing,' but also euthanasia which is *not* voluntary."

According to the *Encyclopedia of Bioethics*,

Until the seventeenth century, "euthanasia" generally referred to any means for an "easy" death; for example, by leading a temperate life or by cultivating an acceptance of mortality. However, upon entering the domain of medicine, with Francis Bacon's *Advancement of Learning* (1605), "euthanasia" increasingly came to connote specifically measures taken by the physician, including the possibility of hastening death. It is the latter meaning of a more rapid death that has been prevalent in the twentieth century, often in reference to the movement to reform legislation for that purpose.[1]

In this chapter we shall see examples of both "active" and "passive" euthanasia. In relating euthanasia to the increasing use of life supports, which it defines as "contingent measures to keep a patient alive who otherwise shortly would die," the *Encyclopedia* continues:

> This development of life support has tended recently to preempt the meaning of "prolongation of life" thereby placing it in contradistinction to euthanasia. Moreover, it has tended to displace the popular import of "euthanasia" from active intervention to a passive withholding of "extraordinary" measures.[2]

In a further definition, active euthanasia is viewed as a situation where "death is actively brought about," whereas passive euthanasia is defined as . . .

> death which comes through the leaving out or neglecting of life-preserving measures. Thus to shoot someone is to commit an act; but to refuse help to the victim of the shooting is an omission . . . distinguished from a "natural" death.[3]

Roots of Discrimination

In the Third Reich, as we have seen earlier, euthanasia started with the killing of Germans as well as non-Germans who were terminally ill, aged, or "defective." Indeed, in order to properly understand euthanasia as it is talked about today, it is essential to look back into the history of German psychiatry, at least as far back as Dr. Emil Kraeplin who lived during the latter part of the nineteenth century, died in 1926, and is generally accepted as the father of modern psychiatry. What is not so generally known, however, is that many also consider him to be the father of Nazism.

Originally, what psychiatrists call "psychosis" had been thought of only in organic terms. That is, when people were psychotic or insane or out of touch with reality it was thought that they were that way because of an obvious physical problem, such as a brain tumor. Emil Kraeplin, however, arrived at theories concerning the causes of vague, so-called mental illnesses, which in themselves had not been proven to even exist—hoping that eventually some organic causes would be demonstrated which would not only show the causes of these diseases but actually prove their very existence.[4] And so psychiatry had added to *organic* psychosis the vague concept of "functional" psychosis. As with abortion today, this development opened a Pandora's box of potential evil. Diseases which often could not be proven to even exist, much less be given a precise cause or a prognosis, became a major tool for committing people against their will, a practice which continues to this day. It is easier to hospitalize people and even kill them under the guise of a loose psychiatric diagnosis which cannot be objectively proven, than to use a more precise medical diagnosis. Thus psychiatry became a tool of the killing process of the Third Reich.

Even in the area of what used to be called feeblemindedness and what today is called mental retardation, the boundaries between normal and abnormal are not as clear as we might like to think they are. IQ tests are culturally influenced, sometimes ineffectively administered and, at best, not precise. I have seen hearing-impaired children test low because no one realized they couldn't hear a good deal of the test. Children who have been abused and kept isolated for years test low because they don't even know what a shell is— or sand, or a beach or an elephant or a train—much less how many weeks there are in a year.

I have seen many children placed in special education classes who should not be there. The result is that a child who is already having problems of one kind or another now feels that his low view of himself is correct.

I was a teacher for thirteen years in both private and

public schools, was also a school counselor during three of those years, and spent an additional three years doing group counseling (mainly related to drug abuse) with high school students. I also started the first class for the emotionally handicapped in a given high school. Many of the students who are in special education classes do not belong there. Often they are "dumped" there because other teachers do not want them in the average classes. Once such a placement occurs, whether or not the placement is appropriate, other students often tease them, call them "stupid" and, in general, isolate them. If the placement is one of "dumping" rather than legitimate academic need, not only do these students get worse in such a placement, but they prevent the few who do need special education from getting the truly specialized help they need.

Would They Have Killed Her?

It is dangerous to believe that labels like retarded, learning disabled, neurotic, hyper-active, even schizophrenic or manic depressive, are some kind of concrete evaluations from God himself. At best they can be useful in defining the kind of help which *might* be prescribed. At worst they stigmatize, isolate and, under certain political regimes, can be the justification for mass extermination.

A few years ago I saw a girl in my office who was sixteen and was entering the tenth grade in classes designed for the mentally retarded. She was from another state and I only saw her two times. Her parents were concerned because of her emotional problems, not because of her academic placement. She had been diagnosed at an early age as mentally retarded by the staff of a prestigious medical institution. She had spent the better part of her school years in classes for the retarded. She looked retarded, she talked as the retarded talk, and she acted in ways which are appropriate to the more severely retarded. Yet as we talked, I had the strange feeling that underneath all of the retarded behavior, this girl was of normal intelligence.

I had her retested rather extensively at the same institution where she had been tested as a small child. I received back an amazing letter. She had normal intelligence, they replied, and had definitely *never* been mentally retarded! But, they said in amazement, she does seem to have some strange behavior. Of course she had strange behavior! She had spent her life with children who had very low intelligence and had learned to act like them. She had learned to play act at being mentally retarded until now she viewed such behavior as normal. After all, it had been normal in her isolated world.

On such a flimsy basis this child would have been killed during the Third Reich. Even in this country she would have been in danger if she had lived in the wrong place at the wrong time.

"Better for All the World!"

The Nazis passed their sterilization law on July 26, 1933, a bill which took effect on January 1, 1934. During that first year, according to the *Journal of the American Medical Association* in a 1935 issue, "It appears that in 1934 a total of 84,525 petitions were filed.... Of these 84,525 petitions, 64,499 were heard before the eugenics courts, and in 56,244 instances sterilization was ordered."[5] While stating that the opposition of the German public was great and was on the increase, the article goes on to explain that the ruling party in Germany had "taken a strong stand against these objectors ..." The journal then quotes from the correspondence column of the National-Socialist party which says: "It is strongly emphasized that the life of a nation takes precedence over dogma and conflicts of conscience."[6]

Earlier in the United States, in 1907, Indiana was the first state to have a sterilization law on its books. By 1933 when the Nazis joined in, the United States had already forcibly sterilized 16,066 people.[7]

The most famous test case was in Virginia, which passed its sterilization law in 1924. A Dr. A. S. Priddy filed a petition for the sterilization of Carrie Buck, an eighteen-year-old who was considered to have a mental age of nine. Her mother as well as the girl's own children were felt to be defective. Dr. Priddy died during the proceedings, and so a Dr. Bell took his place. The case became known as Buck v. Bell.

The case was appealed to the United States supreme court, where Justice Oliver Wendell Holmes upheld the constitutionality of the statute. In his famous opinion, Holmes stated that:

> Whenever the superintendent of certain institutions . . . shall be of the opinion that it is for the best interests of the patients and of society that an inmate under his care should be sexually sterilized, he may have the operation performed upon any patient afflicted with hereditary forms of insanity, imbecility, &c., on complying with the very careful provisions by which the act protects the patients from possible abuse.

Toward the conclusion of his opinion this famous American poet and justice of the Supreme Court of the United States stated:

> It is better for all the world if instead of waiting to execute degenerate offspring for crime, or to let them starve for their imbecility, society can prevent those who are manifestly unfit from continuing their kind. The principle that sustains compulsory vaccination is broad enough to cover cutting the Fallopian tubes.

At the end of Holmes's statement a simple sentence reads: "Mr. Justice Butler dissents." What a historical accolade for Mr. Butler![8]

In the context of the Nazis' goal of eradicating the Jewish race, feeblemindedness and functional psychosis provided catch-all labels which the Nazis used for anyone they wanted to get rid of. They simply were mentally ill or defective and should therefore be committed. It became a short step from hospital confinement to the gas chambers and crematoriums. Ultimately, hospitals were not even used, just concentration camps.

Furthermore, the psychiatry of the day became closely linked to the study of eugenics, or what we would call genetic engineering. Using the loose diagnosis of functional psychosis, Nazi ideologists like Ernst Rudin, student of Kraeplin and founder of the German Society for Racial Hygiene, became fanatical about purifying the human race. Purification to them included the annihilation of the Jews, whom they claimed were more prone to functional psychosis. The machinery was set for the eventual slaughter of six million Jews.

Discussing psychiatry in the Third Reich, researcher Kenneth Asp stated in an interview that: "The big missing piece in all the literature is functional psychosis: where it came from, why it was developed, and its relationship to the euthanasia movement." Continued Asp: "If you don't understand the technical aspects of psychiatry, you'll never understand the modern euthanasia movement at all."[9]

The concept that the Holocaust in Nazi Germany during World War II started with medicalized killing by German psychiatrists is not an unfounded idea nor is it new. But it has remained until recently a little known fact. In *A Sign for Cain*, Dr. Fredric Wertham acknowledges the *positive* role Germany played in the development of modern psychiatry:

> It is a great achievement of psychiatry to have brought about the scientific and humane treatment of mental patients after centuries of struggles against great obstacles. In this progress, as is universally acknowledged, German psychiatrists played a prominent part. And German public psychiatric hospitals had been among the best and most humane in the world.[10]

Yet it was in the psychiatric arena that the medicalized killing began. The process was planned, precise, and massive.

Starting in 1939, psychiatric patients were systematically killed, until the total number of patients left in the psychiatric hospitals of Berlin alone had dropped by three-fourths by 1945.[11] "Useless eaters" like retarded children, the old, and even World War I veterans who had lost a limb were included in the killing process as well. Ironically, however, at the outset, "Jewish mental patients, old and young, were strictly spared and excluded. The reason given was that they did not deserve the 'benefit' of psychiatric euthanasia. This lasted up to the second half of 1940."[12] After that they were almost all killed very rapidly as part of Hitler's genocide.

"Permission to Destroy Life"

The seed for the concept of life unworthy of life was apparently in the German culture even before Hitler made it so famous. As previously noted, in 1920 a jurist, Karl Binding, and a neurologist, Alfred Hoche, published a book entitled *The Permission to Destroy Life Not Worth Living*, in which euthanasia was advocated for those suffering from incurable physical and mental illness, as well as for the severely retarded. In a review in the *Journal of the American Medical Association* written by the Berlin Correspondent and dated 1920, the book is described as advocating the destruction of all those who are incurably insane, "irrespective as to whether the mental disease is of congenital origin or otherwise." Cost and burden of care is given as one reason to kill such people. The review states that the book also advocated the killing of mentally sound people who are incurably ill and wish to end their lives, as well as those in a coma who "would only awaken to indescribable pain and misery." The decision for the life and death of these latter was to be left to the discretion of the state or the attending physician.[13]

Thus the concept of life unworthy of life came into focus in a most prominent way before Hitler rose to power. The book was well received by the German people and was endorsed by Hitler. It became a formative influence on the German people, and perhaps on Hitler himself.

Like today, *cost* was high on the list of criteria for determining medical care during the Third Reich. According to Dr. Alexander:

A widely used high school mathematics text, *Mathematics in the Service of National Political Education*, includes problems stated in distorted terms of the cost of caring for and rehabilitating the chronically sick and crippled. One of the problems asked, for instance, how many new housing units could be built and how many marriage allowance loans could be given to newly wedded couples for the amount of money it cost the state to care for "the crippled, the criminal and the insane."[14]

Again like today, the inherently human desire to take the easy way out helped inspire public approval of Hitler's euthanasia policies. Before Hitler's authorization of euthanasia in the 1920s, many parents already wanted to be able to seek mercy killing for their disabled children. The nation was ready.

It is important to keep in mind that Hitler's authorization for euthanasia was just that: *permission* to kill, not an order to kill. Comments Dr. D. Alan Shewmon:

Significantly, Hitler's authorization was not so much a command but an extension of "the authority of physicians . . . so that a mercy death may be granted to patients who according to human judgment are incurably ill according to the most critical evaluation of the state of their disease.[15]

The *machinery* for medicalized killing was, however, set in precise motion:

All state institutions were required to report on patients who had been ill five years or more and who were unable to work, by filling out questionnaires giving name, race, marital status, nationality, next of kin, whether regularly visited and by whom, who bore financial responsibility and so forth. The decision regarding which patients should be killed was made entirely on the basis of this brief information by expert consultants, most of whom were professors of psychiatry in the key universities. The consultants never saw the patients themselves.[16]

The more direct political orders came later—for the Jews! Meanwhile, some of the people were pleased when Hitler, upon coming to power, took an interest in their dilemmas with "defective" and ill relatives. Euthanasia of mental patients and those considered defective continued until the end of the war, paralleling the process of genocide.

Dr. Wertham gives a poignant example of the euthanasia of children in one of the hospitals in Germany:

In Eglfing-Haar, which had an excellent reputation as a psychiatric hospital, there was a children's division with a capacity of about 150 children called the *kinderhaus*. This division had a "special department" with twenty-five beds and cribs for the children about to be exterminated. In June, 1945, it was still occupied by twenty children. They were saved by the American Army. In the children's "special department" there was a small room. It was bare except for a small white-tiled table. At the window was a geranium plant which was always carefully watered. Four or five times a month a psychiatrist and a nurse took a child to this little room. A little while later they came out alone.[17]

Dr. Wertham states:

The tragedy is that the psychiatrist did not have to have an order. They acted on their own. They were not carrying out a death sentence pronounced by somebody else. They were the legislators who laid down the rules for deciding who was to die; they were the administrators who worked out the procedures, provided the patients and places, and decided the methods of killing; they pronounced a sentence of life or death in every individual case; they were the executioners who carried the sentences out or—without being coerced to do so—surrendered their patients to be killed in other institutions; they supervised and often watched the slow deaths.[18]

These physicians of the Third Reich were not underlings. They were men of prominence. They were leaders of their day. They were heads of medical schools and hospitals. They were the personification of the truth of the statement two centuries ago by Dr. Christoph Hupeland: "If the doctor presumes to take into consideration in his work whether a life has value or not, the consequences are boundless and the physician becomes the most dangerous man in the state."[19]

Yet the psychiatrists of the Third Reich were not inherently more evil than other physicians of their day. Nor, as some would like to assume from this discussion, does psychiatry need to be inherently evil today. But the built-in looseness of diagnosis combined with the current fad then, and again now, to improve the human race by genetic engineering, provided a tool by which evil could prosper. For while genetic engineering, for example, can be used to avoid certain hereditary diseases, it can also be used to attempt to develop a "super race," and to weed out those characteristics and those people who are not wanted by a given society at a given time.

There is little difference between the power available through genetic engineering and psychiatric diagnoses . . . and nuclear fission. All three have great potential for both good and evil. Diseases can be controlled and great human suffering can be eliminated through genetic engineering and psychiatry, and nuclear power can be harnessed for a vast number of positive uses. They are merely tools, not powerful in themselves without human intervention, and certainly not inherently evil. Yet, just as splitting the atom can result in a Hiroshima, so psychiatry and eugenics can result in something like the Nazi Holocaust.

Could It Have Happened Here?

Looking again at the current potential dangers involving the practice of euthanasia, Dr. Shewmon explains:

> The euthanasia propaganda then was essentially no different from what it is now. . . . There was continuing reference to the costs of caring for the handicapped, retarded, and insane. The purpose behind such propaganda was to facilitate the ongoing program of involuntary "euthanasia." But the point here is that—whether voluntary or involuntary—the indications for legalized killing naturally expand. Eventually patients with minor deformities, the mildly senile, amputee war veterans, "problem children," bed-wetters, and the like were being selected by physicians on their own initiative for "mercy deaths."[20]

In Germany the process quickly escalated from so-called mercy killing to those who were just not wanted and eventually to Hitler's long term goal: the attempted annihilation of European Jews. And in the Third Reich euthanasia always remained in the hands of the medical profession; it remained medicalized killing.

The attitude toward medical ethics that existed in Germany was not as isolated to the Third Reich as one might wish to feel. In July 1942, when Germany's program of medicalized murder would have been known to leaders in American psychiatry, the *Journal of the American Psychiatric Association* published two articles debating what amounted to a "final solution" for retarded people in America. In one of the articles Dr. Foster Kennedy advocated laws that would permit the killing of incurably retarded five-year-old children. In the other article, Dr. Leo Kanner, a well-known child psychiatrist, spoke against euthanasia but suggested sterilization as a possible alternative to killing. The *Journal's* editors, discussing the issue, resorted to euphemisms like "disposal by euthanasia" and "merciful passage from life," and recommended an education campaign to prepare the general public for acceptance of euthanasia.

In two particularly chilling statements, Foster Kennedy answered two objections from his opponents. To those who say: "But these creatures have immortal souls," he replied:

> To them I would answer, in all respect and reverence, that to release the soul from its misshapen body which only defeats in this world the soul's powers and gifts is surely to exchange, on that soul's behalf, bondage for freedom.[21]

To the argument that parents would be shocked and hurt, he replied:

> Parents of defective children appeal to us doctors again and yet again that their unhappy offspring be mercifully released from life. When I first wrote on this subject my mail was filled with letters from all parts of this country carrying sad pleas to which the law and the social mores could provide no answer.[22]

I find Dr. Kennedy believable on the accuracy of this last point, although not morally justifiable in his conclusions. I have on several occasions had parents bring a child to see me who had been committed by them to a mental hospital for an average of two to three months. When I asked why a seemingly upset child had been committed to a mental hospital when his or her condition seemed nowhere near warranting such extreme measures, I was told that the decision had been between boarding school or a mental hospital. They chose a mental hospital each time because their insurance would cover it! In one case the mother had a new baby with whom she wanted to spend time, rather than worrying about a rebellious teenager; in another case, the father of the child had just re-married and his new wife gave him an ultimatum between herself and the child. The child lost!

Let me repeat for emphasis: the upset child, the rebellious teen, the child of the remarried father ... had been committed to *mental* institutions!

In wonderful contrast there was the young couple who had decided to adopt an older child who was very emotionally disturbed from past abuse; they were told by their social worker that the child's condition had worsened to the point where she might have to be hospitalized. The prospective parents were asked if they would like to reconsider. "No," the husband replied. "If she has to be hospitalized at least let her be hospitalized with our name so that she'll know we love her and want her. And so that others will know, too."

Medical ethicist, the late Paul Ramsey, testifying a few years ago before a government committee on the future of medical ethics, issued the following warning: "Remote possibilities are soon proximate, and soon done."[23] The events of the Third Reich, and particularly some of the events which prepared the way for the Holocaust, are either not generally known or have become clothed in fiction and sensationalized as pieces of entertainment. Their reality has begun to be blunted by time. But they did happen. Germans as well as other people were killed because they were considered to be life unworthy of life. Jews were killed—six million Jews—just because they were Jews. Ultimately, only a comparatively small number of people were killed because they chose death in order to avoid a painful disease or a hopeless existence. A philosophy which chipped away at the sanctity of life eventuated into a medicalized killing which quickly became involuntary rather than voluntary euthanasia.

It *Is* Happening in Holland

The Netherlands provides a current, graphic example and warning of how quickly a country can change, and how dangerous is that first step toward medicalized killing. In Holland, that land we usually associate with windmills and wooden shoes, active, voluntary euthanasia is not yet legal but it is readily available upon request. According to a 1987 report, in a population of about 14 million, there are five thousand to eight thousand cases of euthanasia each year. The report states, however, that these figures may not show the full picture because sometimes physicians suppress the facts.[24] In addition, according to a study cited in *Euthanasia in the Netherlands* published by H. J. de Roy van Zuydewijn, Secretary to the Health Council, The Hague, 23 March 1987:

> Sixty-eight percent of the population of the Netherlands as a whole and 69 percent of the country's Roman Catholics are in favour of legalizing euthanasia as defined by the State Commission, provided the criteria formulated by the Commission are adhered to.[25]

While euthanasia occurs in other European nations, the Netherlands seems to be the window through which the world is at present viewing the issue.

Addressing the issue of why euthanasia should be performed, Dr. Pieter Admiraal of Delft, Holland, said:

> Real pain never can be a reason. Pain can and has to be treated. But the real reason seldom is pain. It is the suffering for a multitude of reasons which you all can imagine and the details of which I will not elaborate upon here.[26]

In a tragic partial explanation of what might be presumed to be some of those reasons, Jeane Tromp Meesters wrote in *The Euthanasia Review:*

> Approximately a third of our clients are incurably ill, although not all of them in a terminal state. Many of them suffer from cancer. One fifth of the demands for help come from old to very old people who suffer from different kinds of old-age ailments such as loneliness, isolation, or the feeling that they have lived long enough.[27]

If it is true that a nation must judge itself by how it treats the poor and the helpless and the aged, then perhaps some self-examination by all of us would be appropriate. Certainly it would seem mandatory for those of us who claim to possess the love of God. No one should feel so desperate that he or she considers euthanasia because he is homeless, or sick and in need of care, or lonely or just old. Some of us who are

Christians may never have to answer to God for the taking of our own lives. But we may be found more responsible than we had thought we were for the person alongside us who chose death over life because we didn't reach out to help.

> But if any one has this world's wealth and sees that his brother man is in need, and yet hardens his heart against him—how can such a one continue to love God? Dear children, let us not love in words only nor with the lips, but in deed and in truth (1 John 3:17-18, Weymouth).

The "how" of euthanasia in the Netherlands is perhaps even more interesting than the "why." In a sense, the doctors of Holland are above the law; for in spite of the fact that euthanasia is *not* legal in the Netherlands, doctors who practice it "will not be prosecuted provided that they can prove they have followed certain circumscribed guidelines. Such immunity from prosecution applies only to doctors and to no one else."[28] Indeed, in 1984, "the Supreme Court [of the Netherlands] has ruled that a doctor in terminating the life of a patient on his request, may have acted under *force majeure* (conflict of duties)."[29] "*Force majeure*" seems to be the primary defense by which doctors in Holland supervent successful prosecution.

In Holland, as in the United States, the first battles arose over abortion. And, as in the United States, the courts became involved after the fact, so to speak, and either avoided prosecutions and/or sought to pass laws which supported what was already being done in fact. "The Royal Dutch Medical Association has gone as far as endorsing euthanasia upon demand, not only for adults, but for children without parental consent."[30] Following a euthanasia procedure, death certificates are sometimes falsified in order to avoid an awkward investigation; and, according to some witnesses, many of the elderly in Holland do not consult physicians out of fear that they will be killed rather than healed.[31]

In a recent educational television series, "By the Year 2000," aired on station KCET (Los Angeles) July 26, 1989, Dr.

Christopher De Giorgio, neurologist at L. A. County USC Medical Center, stated:

> It's estimated that there are more cases of involuntary euthanasia practiced in the Netherlands than actually voluntary euthanasia. . . . In some emergency rooms . . . there are many cases where the patient comes in, in pulmonary edema—not a terminal illness—say they're over the age of seventy-five—they're given a lethal injection in the emergency room, without their consent, without their knowledge. . . . In the Netherlands, the handicapped, the elderly, are afraid to go to hospitals because they're afraid of involuntary euthanasia.

Dr. Richard Fenigsen, a cardiologist in the Netherlands, reinforces De Giorgio's report:

> Doctors allow at least 300 handicapped newborn Dutch babies to die every year; prevent surgery for congenital heart disease in Down syndrome children by refusing to give anesthesia; and refuse to implant pacemakers for heart block in patients older than seventy-five or to treat acute small pulmonary edema in the elderly and in single people without close family. Some doctors justify these practices by arguing that it is in those patients' own best interests to die as soon as possible, but often the explanation is that society should not be burdened with keeping such persons alive. The decisions are taken without the knowledge of the patients and against their will.[32]

In a country where euthanasia is still technically illegal, according to Dr. Fenigsen, some people feel compelled to carry a card which declares that they do not wish to have euthanasia performed on them.

Dr. Fenigsen attributes the willingness of the Dutch people to submit to the idea of euthanasia in part to . . .

> all-intrusive propaganda in favor of death. The highest terms of praise have been applied to the request to die: this act is "brave," "wise," and "progressive." All efforts are made to convince people that this is what they ought to do, what society expects of them, and what is best for themselves and their families.[33]

Dr. Fenigsen makes a dire prediction for the Netherlands if euthanasia is actually legalized, a prediction which other countries cannot afford to ignore:

> Proposals calling for euthanasia of handicapped newborns mean that doctors acting, as they do everywhere, under state supervision, will issue some newborn citizens permits to live and destroy others. To exist, a human being will have to be approved by the government—a reversal of the democratic principle that governments, to exist, have to be approved by people.[34]

The sad irony of Holland lies in its history during World War II. When, in 1941, the physicians of Holland were ordered by the Nazis to focus their medical attention on those who could be used for labor in the Reich, and to turn in questionnaires on patients' health, Holland refused. The order was subtle and did not state its aims clearly. But Dutch doctors saw through the well-phrased words and they detected a first step toward medicalized killing. The questionnaires which they refused to fill out and turn in did, indeed, turn out to be a primary tool used in the identification and killing of those considered unworthy of life according to the Reich. The Dutch doctors were then threatened with their jobs, at which time they returned their licenses and saw their patients in secret—with no paper work.

According to Dr. Alexander, Arthur Seyss-Inquart, Reich commissar for the Occupied Netherlands Territories, then . . .

> retraced his steps and tried to cajole them—still to no effect. Then he arrested 100 Dutch physicians and sent them to concentration camps. The medical profession remained adamant and quietly took care of their widows and orphans, but would not give in. Thus it came about that not a single euthanasia or non-therapeutic sterilization was recommended or participated in by any Dutch physician. They had the foresight to resist before the first step was taken, and they acted unanimously and won out in the end.[35]

Yet at the time of the writing of this book, Holland is in the forefront in the practice of euthanasia, the example to the world, even as it was the example to the world in its stand against euthanasia during World War II.

Eliminate Suffering . . .
Or Eliminate the Patient?

Nor do the horror stories of our time exclude the United States. Prenatal decisions define quality of life for an unborn being who never has the chance to be born and discover his own meaning in life. Unwanted babies are starved and allowed to die in some of our hospitals. "Mercy killings" are often not prosecuted. We are beginning to *talk* like a nation which is preparing for the acceptance of euthanasia. We kill the unborn with nothing more than regret. Quality of life has become a household term. We base medical treatment of our loved ones on what we imagine they would want, rather than in terms of right and wrong. Has it become so old fashioned to call something wrong that we can't even include the concept of sin in our discussions of something as important as the taking of a human life?

For historically, voluntary euthanasia has almost always, if not always, turned from voluntary to involuntary, from the relief of pain to the freeing of society of those who have become unwanted. Rationalizations, like "I know this is what she would have wanted," and "He never wanted to end up like this," salve the conscience.

In referring to the Third Reich Dr. Alexander aptly observed:

> Whatever proportions these crimes finally assumed, it became evident to all who investigated them that they had started from small beginnings. The beginnings at first were merely a subtle shift in emphasis in the basic attitude of the physicians. It started with the acceptance of the attitude, basic in the euthanasia movements, that there is such a thing as life not worthy to be

lived. This attitude in its early stages concerned itself merely with the severely and chronically sick. Gradually the sphere of those to be included in this category was enlarged to encompass the socially unproductive, the ideologically unwanted, the racially unwanted and finally all non-Germans. But it is important to realize that the infinitely small wedged-in lever from which this entire trend of mind received its impetus was the attitude toward the nonrehabilitable sick.

According to this standard, we in the free world are already where the Third Reich was not long before the atrocities began!

Continued Dr. Alexander in his very valuable and often quoted 1949 article:

> It is, therefore, this subtle shift in emphasis of the physicians' attitude that one must thoroughly investigate. It is a recent significant trend in medicine including psychiatry, to regard prevention as more important than cure. Observations and recognition of early signs and symptoms have become the basis for prevention of further advance of disease.[36]

Preventative medicine, while commendable in itself, can feed into a tendency to join with eugenics in its emphasis on preserving those who are strong and restoring them to productivity, as well as protecting the genetic material, rather than comforting and maintaining the physically weak. Such an emphasis in medicine can prepare doctors, as it did in the Third Reich, to identify the "weak" and the "defective" and select them out for so-called mercy killing, or, at best, sterilization.

Biologist Leon Kass points out the danger of depersonalizing the patient by referring to him by his disease rather than emphasizing his personhood. From the point of view of genetic abortion, Kass asks the question:

> For in the case of what other disease does preventive medicine consist in the elimination of the patient at risk? . . . A person is more than his disease. And yet we slide easily from the language

of possession to the language of identity, from "he has hemophilia" to "he is a hemophiliac," from "she has diabetes" through "she is diabetic" to "she is a diabetic," from "the fetus had Down's syndrome" to "the fetus is a Down's." This way of speaking encourages the belief that it is defective persons (or potential persons) that are being eliminated, rather than diseases.[37]

Kass presents a telling quote from Abraham Lincoln which aptly applies whenever we begin to think that someone, unborn or born, does not have the right quality of life to be left alive. It shows once again the ridiculous extremes to which certain perverted logic can be extended. Furthermore, it illustrates the possibility that once you deem someone not worthy of life or freedom, the pathway by which you arrived at such a conclusion can easily turn back on you. It has some application as well to the danger of using the knowledge of preventive medicine as a tool to predict who is worthy of life:

If A. can prove, however conclusively, that he may, of right, enslave B.—why may not B. snatch the same argument, and prove equally, that he may enslave A?

You say A. is white, and B. is black. It is *color*, then; the lighter, having the right to enslave the darker? Take care. By this rule, you are to be slave to the first man you meet, with a fairer skin than your own.

You do not mean *color* exactly? You mean the whites are *intellectually* the superiors of the blacks, and, therefore have the right to enslave them? Take care again. By this rule, you are to be slave to the first man you meet, with an intellect superior to your own.

But, say you, it is a question of *interest*; and, if you can make it your *interest*, you have the right to enslave another. Very well. And if he can make it his interest, he has the right to enslave you.[38]

So it will be with euthanasia. It will never stop with simple mercy killing at the request of the terminal patient. Furthermore, it has the potential to join with genetic engineering in a quest to purify the race—a term which still rings in our collective memory! If that happens it will be used to get rid of anyone whom anyone in power cares to be rid of. It will ultimately turn on the very people who supported it. The intellectually bright will not be considered bright any longer. The once healthy will no longer be healthy enough to be truly productive. Once again it will be a patriotic duty to eliminate the "cancer" from the organism called society—whoever we consider the cancer at that time. But what will be left will be a national, or global, moral character which will be evil and rotten from within.

In practical terms involuntary euthanasia would not be that difficult to facilitate. It is human nature to deceive people into doing something we want them to do when we know that they may resist it if we tell them the truth. While such deceit may go against our moral character, the pangs of conscience are easily assuaged if the person to be deceived is very old, or very young, or mentally defective, or someone we don't respect.

Last year a young woman related to me how her family had "convinced" her grandmother to go into a convalescent home. The elderly lady was told that she needed to go there "for a few days" because her doctor "wanted her to get extra rest and treatment." Grumbling a little, the older lady agreed, "as long as it wasn't too many days." Relieved at her compliance, the family assured her that she could come home "when she was better," a time which, of course, never came! In their minds the lie was a small one. After all, they reasoned, maybe she *would* get better.

The elderly, the sick, and the very young are often dealt with in this way. And at times it can seem humane. The problem is that eventually they catch on to the deceit and the disillusionment is greater than ever.

What About Uncle Joe?

It is not inconceivable that the following situation could occur in the not so distant future: There could be a family of six—a mother and father with two teenage children, an elderly grandparent and an Uncle Joe who was getting up in years and had, therefore, moved in with the family after the death of his wife. In years past, Uncle Joe was fast-living and hard-drinking, but so full of wit and good humor that no one minded his shortcomings. When he was drunk, he went to sleep. And besides all that, he worked hard during the day, made a good salary and thus was a financial help to the family.

Times were changing, however. The family needed the money less now. With the father's salary increases life had become relatively easy. More than that, Uncle Joe had ceased to be fun. Rather than sleeping off his drinking bouts, he shouted and demanded. Furthermore, he was moving toward the age of retirement when no one relished the idea of having him home all the time. The children, too, were no longer small and pliable, and the mother needed an extra room for crafts. Uncle Joe had changed. The family had changed. And nobody wanted him in his old age.

Even a convalescent home was no longer an option. The government didn't pay for that anymore. And it seemed a shame to waste Uncle Joe's life savings when his quality of life was so poor anyway. Uncle Joe, as they had known him, wouldn't want that! Furthermore, the children needed that extra money for college.

One day the father would ask Uncle Joe to go with him to the doctor's office. Uncle Joe, not being entirely cantankerous, would go, just to keep the father company. While at the doctor's office the father could have a brief consultation with the doctor regarding Uncle Joe. A few papers would be signed, and Uncle Joe would be persuaded to have a flu shot. Then the father would return home, *alone*.

It wouldn't be that hard to do, with the right mind set.

After all, why doom a nice man like Uncle Joe to an alcoholic's death? Didn't we do as much for the family dog last year?

"A Bodyguard of Lies"

There are, however, times when deceit could conceivably be used in a positive way. Those who operated as forces of the Resistance in World War II, for example, often had great conflict over the need to lie if they were to save human lives. These were not lies of convenience, nor were the people who lied individuals who were used to deceit. For the most part they were the best of the population. They were people with courage and conviction.

Those in the Resistance, and particularly those who were Christians and wanted to help the Jews, were confronted with two biblical commandments: "Thou shalt not kill," and, "Thou shalt not lie." There was no way for anyone involved to avoid making the decision of which one to obey. To make no decision was to decide by default. To decide not to save a life because it involved telling a lie was to become responsible for that life being taken by someone else.

Using a lie as a weapon for good is a very dangerous undertaking spiritually. The Bible teaches the principle of truth. In Deuteronomy 32:4 we read that God is a "God of truth." We are told in Psalm 91:4 that "His truth shall be thy shield and buckler." Certainly for the Christian, truth is to be a principle of our lives.

Yet as we look at recent history we recall a godly lady in Holland by the name of Corrie ten Boom who hid Jewish people from the SS and lied about their whereabouts, faked passports, used illegal food ration cards and employed every type of deception in order to protect right. In a meeting of the Allies in 1943, Winston Churchill made the comment that, "In wartime, truth is so precious that she should always be attended by a bodyguard of lies."[39]   The remark was translated for Stalin, who chuckled. But with those words a unique alliance was struck: the British, American, Russian—and, in part, the German—secret services would now be united in a plan to rid the world of Hitler. Surely Churchill would have also believed that Corrie ten Boom's cause was so precious that it, too, needed to be protected by a "bodyguard of lies."

The Scriptures themselves seem to back up Miss ten Boom. In Joshua 2, for example, when Rahab lied in order to protect the two Israelite spies, she was rewarded by God. In verse 14 when Rahab asked that the lives of her family be spared, she was told: "Our life for yours, if ye utter not our business." Since she had already been asked specifically about their whereabouts, it seems unlikely that she could continue to hide what she knew without actual deceit.

Another biblical example of God-inspired deceit is in Exodus where the midwives of Egypt were told to kill every boy-child delivered of an Israelite woman. The midwives disobeyed that order. Furthermore, when they were later questioned about the large numbers of male children being born, they lied and claimed that Hebrew women tended to have their children before the mid-wives arrived (see Exodus 1:20-21). Some might argue that God rewarded them in spite of what they did. But God doesn't reward sin, and so one has to conclude that this deception, and that of Rahab, were deceptions which were used to protect righteousness. They were part of that arsenal of words which, in these instances, were used to bodyguard the truth.

As a Christian who is fully aware of the biblical regard for truth, I hesitate to talk about exceptions. Yet throughout the history of the church we have been confronted with the dilemma of whether or not it is ever right to deal in untruth. Someday many of us may be faced with moral dilemmas where we will need to have thought this issue out before those dilemmas arise. Someone's life may depend on whether we hide them or whether we turn them over to an evil power because we fear to lie.

Returning once again to Le Chambon and Magda Trocme, author Philip Hallie, in his book about the village says:

> To this day, Magda remembers her reaction to hearing about the making of the first counterfeit card. During that first winter of the Occupation, Theis came into the presbytery and said to her, "I have just made a false card for Monsieur Levy. It is the only way to save his life." She remembers the horror she felt at that moment: duplicity, for any purpose, was simply wrong. She and the other leaders knew that ration cards were as important as identity cards—the Chambonnais were so poor that they could not share their food with refugees and hope to survive themselves. Nonetheless, none of those leaders became reconciled to making counterfeit cards, though they made many of them in the course of the Occupation. Even now, Magda finds her integrity diminished when she thinks of those cards. She is still sad over what she calls "our lost candor."[40]

In the Old Testament cities of refuge the inhabitants of the cities were responsible for the physical safety of those entrusted to their care. If a refugee was harmed, those in the city were declared guilty. They were guilty even though they themselves had not performed the act of violence. They were guilty because they had not sufficiently protected the person committed to their care.

Since Le Chambon was patterned after those cities of refuge, the result of not lying would have literally been to assume the guilt of the death of each Jew who sought their protection and was then killed.

In relating these issues back to the overall principle of the sanctity of human life, regardless of laws which would diminish the worth of life and even be in conflict with its existence, Dr. Alexander asks a striking question:

> Should we submit to the capriciousness of temporary-temporal political laws, or stick to our immutable laws of medical ethics? It is my firm belief that the latter outranks the former, as Divine law outranks governmental law, a fact unanimously established by the Nuremberg War Crimes Court.[41]

In the treatment of human beings, a government cannot morally decide who shall live and who shall die, and when. The world has been that way before.

When two general biblical commandments or two biblical principles are in conflict because of a unique set of circumstances, one must either actively choose one commandment over the other . . . or choose passively, by default. To do nothing about either making or not making a false ration card, for example, is to choose by default to allow a certain number of people to starve. On a more immediate level, to hide a person whose life is being threatened and then to refuse to protect him by telling the would-be murderer that he is not in your house, is to choose to be responsible for his death.

When such a dilemma arises, as it well may in some of our lifetimes, we don't create it. It thrusts itself upon us much as it did upon the quiet village of Le Chambon, and a choice must be made, either actively or passively. Those involved in the sanctuary movement in this country have experienced the moral dilemma of lying. Someday, if euthanasia becomes mandatory in certain cases, it is conceivable that we may be asked to hide the elderly, or the defective. When we are asked about their whereabouts, our answer might have to be a blatant, "Grandma doesn't live here anymore," when she's really hiding in the attic.

When my aunt Lydia was dying in the hospital and I was asked if I wanted a "no code," my first reaction was, "This shouldn't be my decision. I just won't make it mine." But it *was* my choice. In the absence of any other family members, I was the only one to make the choice. I could run from it, as I wanted to. But by running, others less qualified would make the choice for me; and by running I would become responsible for their choice. More than that, if no one made a choice, no choice would become an automatic decision to do all the heroics. Again the choice would be made by default, and I would still have been responsible.

God never asks us to do evil that good may come. The

end still does not justify the means. But just as war is the exception to the commandment not to kill, and having a mortgage on a house is an exception to the commandment to owe no man anything, so at times the truth is best safeguarded by a bodyguard of lies. To see this is to enable a reversal, a change in the direction of our behavior, which, while it seems to go contrary to what we would usually do, actually goes in the same direction.

It is in the grey areas ethically, which in particular accompany the fast growth in medical technology, where many of us will fail in our love to each other. We as Christians like our rules to be clear-cut. "Black and white" ethics make us feel safe. But when we enter areas like alternate reproductive techniques and refusal of treatment, there are many grey areas. There are questions for which we do not have ready answers, and there are answers which may vary in their correctness from person to person. These grey areas become an arena for the display of love to our fellow man in general as well as to those who are our brothers and sisters in Christ. These grey areas may well be the greatest test in the twenty-first century of our willingness to love as Christ loved.

For the Christian, while there will be grey areas, there will always be the guidance of God. For it is an absolute promise of God's Word that he will never leave us without a knowledge of his will. That will of God as interpreted by the individual Christian can, for example, integrate the principle of total truth and transparency before God, on the one hand, with the enablement of a bodyguard of lies, on the other hand, in order to obey the commandment of God not to kill. An intimate knowledge of the will of God can, for example, lead a Corrie ten Boom to hide Jews and lie to the Gestapo. It can lead a village like Le Chambon to take in the stranger at their gate and falsify ration cards in order to obey the commandment, "Thou shalt not kill." If killing in self defense is permitted by God, then why not lying? Yet some who would pull a trigger on a murderer who was actively choking out the life of a small child, would hesitate to save that same child by lying about her whereabouts. Let us at least be consistent in our morality!

To do the will of God must be the unchanging principle of our life, not what we feel or even what we consider most loving. We must carry out that will of God in a loving manner, but we can rarely determine morality by just love alone. The righteousness of God and the love of God must be kept in balance if we are to do the will of God. Only by a continual settling down into the will of God can we be sure that when we feel compelled to practice deceit, it will be in the name of Almighty God rather than in the service of evil.

Immortal Until Our Work Is Done

Euthanasia is not without its appeal. While those of us who are Christians have a confidence regarding our eternal destiny, most of us do not relish the idea of how we may die. While the destination may be sure, how we may get there is not!

I can echo the words of C. S. Lewis when he said: "You would like to know how I behave when I am experiencing pain, not writing books about it. You need not guess, for I will tell you; I am a great coward. . . ."[42] When he was asked how a good God could allow suffering, Lewis continued aptly: "What do people mean when they say, 'I am not afraid of God because I know He is good?' Have they never even been to a dentist?"[43]

Dying, as well as living, can be painful and uncomfortable. But it may also be the supreme moment of our lives as far as our relationship with God is concerned. Who knows what worship goes up to God in those last moments? Who can conceive of the "soul work" which may be accomplished in those last days of life? And who can doubt the wisdom of the timing of God? Will not the God of all the earth do right, even in our dying? Did he not love us so much that he sent his only Son to die for our sins? Did not Christ weep in love over Israel, longing to gather them into his arms? May not even one second of our time on this earth be precious to him?

We need to recapture the spirit of bygone years when, even in situations where the physician could not heal (which was perhaps most of the time), he had finely developed the art of comforting. We need to turn from our total emphasis on the technology of medicine back to the *art* of medicine.

I am reminded of the physician Dr. Viktor Frankl, himself an inmate of the death camps, when he stayed behind from what could have been his own possible release in order to minister to a dying patient whom he knew he could not save but he could comfort. I am reminded of people in Auschwitz who valued life so much that they did not run into the wire and take the easier way out, but remained alive, by choice, in a living hell, out of a slim chance that the Allies would deliver them.

Above all, I am reminded of a statement I once heard: "A servant of God is immortal until his work is done." The statement is a challenge to all of us. It is a comfort to those who fear, in some way, the timing of their death. And it is a severe warning to those who feel that they may become gods and determine the life span of either themselves or anyone else; for it is a fearful thing indeed to tamper with God's immortal work.

EIGHT

In His Time

During the year in which my maternal grandfather died, a major flu epidemic took the lives of thousands of other people as well. Unlike some, my grandfather did not die immediately. Rather, his condition gradually worsened over a period of several months.

At that time penicillin had not been discovered, and rather than worrying about over-treatment, the average doctor simply treated to the utmost of his skill with the available technology. Medical ethics were still relatively simple.

My mother's family was a godly one. They lived on a farm in Wisconsin, not far from the famous Wisconsin Dells. Their house was the stopping place for traveling preachers; and they lived there at a time when hospitality still meant feeding an occasional Indian who came trading his goods for a noon meal.

It was natural, therefore, that the family would pray fervently for the recovery of this husband and father who was only in his late fifties. My mother was eighteen at the time and had already experienced a close death when her older sister died giving birth to her first child. It is particularly understandable, therefore, that the thought of losing her father just two years later was overwhelming. Her prayers were insistent upon his healing.

As the months went on and she watched her father suffer she had mixed feelings of wanting him to live and yet not wishing to prolong his suffering. Then came the evening early in the autumn when my mother went outside in order to be alone. Quietly she relinquished her father to the will of God. She did not plead with God to either heal him or take him—just to do his will. When she came back in the house her father was gone. He was with God, in God's time.

Dealing with illness and dying has never been easy. It hurts to lose a loved one, and most of us cling tenaciously to our own finite lives. As we approach the twenty-first century, however, we face medical dilemmas which my grandfather never had to even think about in his lifetime. Modern technology with its many-faceted options has presented us with choices which most of us feel unqualified to make. How far should we treat? When is it right to turn off a respirator? Should certain treatment, like dialysis, be unavailable to certain groups of people, like the aged? Should the availability of certain treatments be based on cost? Should feeding tubes be used for a comatose patient? Should a baby with Down's Syndrome be given life-saving surgery for an unrelated problem? How much chemotherapy or radiation treatment is enough? What about the harvesting of fetal tissue, which is less prone to rejection than that of an adult, and is therefore desirable in the treatment of certain diseases? And, above all, how can we be sure that we are treating the living process rather than merely prolonging the dying process? For Dr. Matthew Conolly, professor of medicine and pharmacology at UCLA School of Medicine, aptly comments that "to prolong the process of dying, or to resuscitate the terminally ill so that they may have the doubtful privilege of dying twice, would be grotesque."[1]

The list of possible medical dilemmas is endless and ever-increasing. A basic principle which can be supported by biblical teaching in resolving some of these difficulties would be to treat life wherever possible and to re-learn the art of comforting the dying. To neglect the treatment of those who could respond while, at the same time, you needlessly extend the process of dying for others, is not only a misuse of modern technology but is to function outside the biblical view of sanctity of life. This is especially true in those cases where scientific experimentation rather than immediate patient care is the goal.

"What is the value of human life?" is a fundamental issue in considering the treatment of life as an obligation. Many people who are very militantly against abortion are not nearly as concerned about the homeless who die in the streets or the aged who die neglected and untreated. There is a tendency in all of us to value life within the perspective of what life we think is important, be it the unborn, the elderly, the handicapped or, more selfishly, just our own life or that of a loved one.

The Sanctity of *All* Human Life

In the Bible there is a consistent thread throughout the Old and New Testaments which emphasizes the sanctity of *all* human life, and, indeed, a respect for even animal life. In Exodus 20:13 the command is simple: "Thou shalt not kill." In Numbers 35:33 (NIV) we read: "Do not pollute the land where you are. Bloodshed pollutes the land. . . ."

Genesis 9:5-6 reads:

> And surely your blood of your lives will I require; at the hand of every beast will I require it, and at the hand of man; at the hand of every man's brother will I require the life of man. Whoso sheddeth man's blood, by man shall his blood be shed: for in the image of God made he man.

In biblical exegesis repetition always has significance. In this case the repetition could well be an emphasis on the importance which God places on human life. Why? Because of the reason given in these verses—that human beings are created in *his* image. A German rabbi, Jacob Mecklenburg, in a book written in Hebrew and not translated into English, comments that there are two ways of killing: One out of hatred, and one out of brotherly love—mercy killing. In his opinion these verses affirm both meanings and, of course, condemn killing for either reason. Whether or not the rabbi is correct in the specific interpretation of this verse, his comments seem in general to be valid; and they are supportive of the biblical view that to kill is wrong, even if the motive be one of kindness.

In his excellent commentary on the Book of Genesis, Arthur Pink says:

> Now, after the flood, capital punishment as the penalty of murder *is* ordained, ordained by God himself, ordained centuries before the giving of the Mosaic law, and therefore, universally binding until the end of time. It is important to observe that the *reason* for this law is not here based upon the well-being of man, but is grounded upon the basic fact that man is made "in the image of God." This expression has at least a twofold significance—a natural and a moral. The moral image of God in man was lost at the Fall, but the natural has been preserved, as is clear from 1 Corinthians 11:7 and James 3:9. It is primarily because man is made in the image of God that it is sinful to slay him.[2] "To deface the King's image is a sort of treason among men, implying a hatred against him, . . . How much more treasonable, then, it must be to destroy, curse, oppress, or in any way abuse the image of the King of Kings!"[3]

Earthly monarchs stamp their images on coins and statues, and those images are respected. The image of a king is not to be desecrated. How awesome to realize that the King of Kings has imprinted his image on his creation, *Man!* This imprint distinguishes man from the rest of the animal world. It, too, is not to be desecrated. We are created in his image and we have been given immortal souls.

A story we read in 1 Samuel 31:3-4 underscores the great worth God places on human life:

> The battle went sore against Saul [the king of Israel], and the archers hit him; and he was sore wounded of the archers. Then said Saul unto his armourbearer, Draw thy sword, and thrust me through therewith; lest these uncircumcised come and thrust me through, and abuse me. But his armourbearer would not; for he was sore afraid. Therefore Saul took a sword, and fell upon it.

Here was a good case for mercy killing if ever there was one. Saul was truly dying. He was in dire pain on a battlefield with no resources for soothing that pain. His enemies were near and might well have tortured him while he was still alive. But his armourbearer, who truly cared about him, would still not kill him.

Later (2 Samuel 1), a man came to David to tell him of the death of Saul. In telling his story the man claimed to have performed euthanasia on Saul, which, of course, was a lie, probably told in order to ingratiate himself with David, who would be the next king. After claiming that Saul had asked to be killed, the man went on to explain: "I stood upon him, and slew him, because I was sure that he could not live after that he was fallen" (2 Samuel 1:9-10).

After a period of mourning, David said to the man: "How wast thou not afraid to stretch forth thine hand to destroy the Lord's anointed?" (v. 14). David then had the man killed, "for thy mouth hath testified against thee, saying, 'I have slain the Lord's anointed'" (v. 16).

And let us not forget that, although the young man had lied about actually killing Saul, it was true that Saul had asked for someone to kill him. He had asked for mercy killing. He had pleaded for euthanasia. But David did not consider that a reason to spare the young man from punishment. Saul's request for a merciful death was wrong and was not to be given in to, either out of hate or out of pity and love.

To refuse mercy killing out of a fear of God may be an unpopular concept in our day, but it is a biblical one. When I was a teenager I went to a Christian high school for several years, and the school verse was Proverbs 9:10: "The fear of the Lord is the beginning of wisdom: and the knowledge of the holy is understanding." From constant repetition the verse became ingrained into my subconscious. Today as I was writing this chapter I realized anew how much we need this concept of fearing God. In a day when we make a cosmic "pal" out of God, it is good to remember that he is God Almighty and that as such his authority is to be unquestioned in the life of the believer.

"Lord, Let Me Die!"

In his book *Facing Death and the Life After*, Billy Graham aptly points out:

> "Lord, let me die," is a prayer and a plea offered to God by many throughout the ages. Moses was not ill, but he was grieved about the burden the Lord had given him. He looked at his people grumbling about their food and their living conditions, complaining until Moses must have reached his limit. He'd had it. He said to God, "If this is how you are going to treat me, put me to death right now" (Numbers 11:5).
>
> But the Lord was not finished with Moses yet! He went on to lead his people through the wilderness and to the boundaries of the Promised Land.
>
> Elijah had killed the prophets of Baal, yet when the evil Queen Jezebel swore she was going to get even, the fearless Elijah ran into the wilderness, sat down under a juniper tree, and cried out, "I have had enough, Lord," he said. "Take my life; I am no better than my ancestors" (1 Kings 19:4).
>
> But the Lord sent an angel to supply him with food and water; essential ingredients for life!
>
> The Lord was not finished with Elijah yet.
>
> And think about Job. He had boils all over his body. His flesh was eaten by worms. His skin was oozing and decaying like rotten turnips. He was so shriveled and thin that his bones were sticking out and he had gnawing pains and frightening dreams. Under such circumstances, most of us would cry out, as Job did, "that God would be willing to crush me, to loose his

hand and cut me off!" (Job 6:9).

But the Lord was not finished with Job yet, either.

If we had been with Job in his pain-wracked, miserable situation, would we have taken away his food and water, and allowed him to starve and dehydrate?[4]

Certainly we would have said that Job had poor *quality of life*. The Nazis would have declared him to be *life unworthy of life*. They would have killed him, for he would not have been fit for even a few pitiful weeks of slave labor! A recent article in the *New England Journal of Medicine*, March 30, 1989, could have conceivably included Job in its definition of candidates for "rational suicide."[5]

The authority of God in matters of life and death is a consistent theme throughout the Bible. God will openly shorten the life of the man who commits murder: "bloody and deceitful men shall not live out half their days" (Psalm 55:23). Even though David was the only man God ever called a "man after his own heart," he was still deprived of his life-goal of building the temple because he had "shed much blood" (1 Chronicles 22:8).

The Christian is dissuaded from euthanasia not only by God's *authority over* life, but also by his *concern for* life. In Psalm 139, where we have previously seen the magnificent care and concern God has for the unborn, we see also his more general care for all human life. W. Graham Scroggie translates verse 3 as: "My path and my couch thou hast winnowed, subjecting all my life to the closest investigation, and art thoroughly familiar with all my ways."[6]

In his commentary on these words Scroggie explains:

Henry Ward Beecher has said: "Before men we stand as opaque bee-hives. They see the thoughts go in and out of us, but what work they do inside of a man they cannot tell. Before God we are as glass bee-hives, and all that our thoughts are doing within us He perfectly sees and understands."[7]

This is a particularly comforting thought for those who are

locked into themselves by paralysis or even a mechanical means like a respirator—that God sees all our thoughts! Someone hears and understands. Someone is in there with us!

Once when I had surgery, right before I was given the general anaesthesia, the pre-op drug caused me to stop breathing, and I became totally paralyzed. I could think, but I couldn't move, and I had no sense of feeling. I have never experienced greater suffering. I felt as if I couldn't endure another moment of the tremendous feeling of pressure in my lungs and the need for air. For some illogical reason, I desperately wished that I could at least choke and move and fight for air. But all I could do instead was think.

First I prayed for life. Then, convinced that I would die, I prayed for unconsciousness. But the one awareness which pervaded the whole experience was that which I had of the reality and presence of God. I have never felt so isolated from earth in my life. But I have never been more sure of the reality of God and of my relationship with him. When all else was cut off, God was there. Since that day I have never doubted that when I die, I will not die alone. God will be with me. For a few moments on that operating table, earth receded and heaven became the greatest reality I knew. Then once again I began to feel. A flicker of air slipped through into my lungs, and I moved; and life on earth was once again more real to me than heaven.

Scroggie continues in his commentary on Psalm 139:

Our path and our couch are known to God; that is, our public and private life; our life by day and by night; our social and secret life. These outward and inward experiences of ours God winnows, discerning what in them is good, and what is bad; taking cognizance of what is chaff and what is wheat with unerring precision and justice; and so all our ways are before Him.[8]

As I got deeper into writing this book, I found myself agonizing over the "what ifs" of possible medical situations which could be painful. While I could never justify any kind of direct euthanasia, it became easy to allow my view of the great value God puts on life to slowly erode, piece by piece. My definition of death veered away from total brain death to cerebral death (in which state bodily functions remain, even though cognitive functions have ceased). And I began to broaden my view of when an individual person could refuse treatment. After all, it is easy to write about noble standards of sanctity of life. But when it's your daughter who's raped and she wants an abortion, or when it's your body that's trapped inside the confines of a respirator, or when it's your body that suffers the ravage of chemotherapy—at such a time any of us might cry out for relief from discomfort, even at the cost of life itself.

Such feelings of desperation are normal. Even Christ evidenced a fear of pain when he prayed in the Garden of Gethsemane. He sweat great drops of blood and prayed that, if possible, "this cup" would pass from him.

"Every Second of Life Is an Opportunity"

In God's perfect timing I had an interview with Rabbi Yitzchok Adlerstein, director of Jewish Studies at Yeshiva University of Los Angeles. I came away with a renewed sense of how precious each moment of a human life is to God. "If a whole life is infinitely valuable," said the rabbi, "then any part of human life is valuable...." He continued:

> In my tradition, every second of life is an opportunity to do another Mitzvah, another commandment. You can do commandments while you are lying in bed without the ability to move, respond or do anything but the conscious linking of your mind to God.... Who can say that, while the patient is in pain and suffering to the extreme, what he is enduring at that moment cannot be something positive for his soul?

To the objection of some that perhaps survival would not

be worth their pain, even if, in the end, they got their life back, he replied:

> What would you tell the people in Auschwitz who thought, "Well, there's a tiny chance that the Germans will lose this war and in a couple of years the Russians and British and Americans will come and we'll still be alive." These inmates might say, "But do you know what I'm experiencing in the meantime? It's not worth it!"

Then looking directly at me, he asked: "Well, is it worth it or isn't it worth it?"

At the suggestion that anyone should relieve another person of pain by shortening their life, the rabbi replied that such action would be "a way of invalidating any significance that the last months or years might otherwise have ... [if you do that] you're creating God in your own image. ..." In his words, the appropriate response to God can only be, "'Look, God, I will go as far as you make me go!' It's not for us to say: 'God, you made a mistake, and we're going to do your work for you and take this person and put him in your arms a little earlier than you had decided.'"

Furthermore, lest we wish that we had been born in an earlier time without the complex dilemmas of modern medical technology, Rabbi Adlerstein concluded:

> God himself presides over you in history and allows you the knowledge that he wants you to have and thinks is appropriate for you and for every generation. Every generation and every time and every city and every place and every human being has his own set of tests and circumstances. ... The environment that I'm in is the one that's best for my personal trip.[9]

Through my conversation with Rabbi Adlerstein the Lord spoke deeply about my own need for renewal in the area of submission to God even in that which is unexplainable and unpleasant. Submission is not a popular word among many of us Christians. We like to "explain" God and then have him function according to our explanations of what he should do. In my office I hear words like, "I'm angry at God because he took away my loved one," or, "I doubt God's goodness because I never seem to get ahead like everyone else does." But throughout man's history God has always combined his love and his knowledge in his dealings with man. Sometimes he loves us enough to let us hurt, and sometimes he loves us enough to remove the hurt. The reason why he allows painful circumstances often remains unknowable. Yet we are never truly content until we submit to him alone for our ultimate protection. Indeed, no other support is safe.

The words of an old song, "Submission," were influential in my teenage years: "I conquer only where I yield." The paradox struck me even then. Like most teenagers, I was into having my own way. But way down inside, I wanted the will of God more. Most Christians are like that. We want freedom from pain and we desire earthly comfort. These are not wrong desires. But deep down, we must want God more; and we must know that we conquer only where we yield.

There is a particular irony in the New Testament treatment of sanctity of life where, *because* life is so precious, we are told that, "Whosoever will save his life shall lose it: and whosoever will lose his life for my sake shall find it." Only when something is established as valuable can it be an appropriate sacrifice to God. If human life is valuable, then to give it back to its Maker is an appropriate, sacrificial gift. If, on the other hand, human life can be thrown away by the caprice of man's desire, then it does not have much value when it is given back to God.

Similarly, the principle of "thou shalt not kill" is fulfilled with an even higher standard in the New Testament. John 15:13 reads: "Greater love hath no man than this, that a man lay down his life for his friends." The sanctity of life here is extended so that, paradoxically, each human life is worth the payment of another life. The worth of this life which God has made in his image is enhanced by the price which may be demanded in order to save it.

The only motivation which could conceivably cause a man to give his own life in order to save the life of another would be love. The supreme example of this is in the voluntary giving up of the divine life of Christ for the human life of each individual person. Divine life was given for human life in the highest example of the worth of man. And the fact that eternal life is promised to man, once again, demonstrates the high valuation God puts on human life.

This giving up of one's life for another is, however, never to be a casual thing. For instance, refusing life-saving treatment so that your children can use the money to buy a new house would not be putting the kind of valuation on human life which is exhibited in Scripture. Indeed, you would be bartering with a life which bears the imprint of God Almighty.

On the other hand, when those university students in Munich who called themselves the White Rose walked into their interrogation sessions, each protecting the lives of the others by claiming to be solely responsible for spreading anti-Nazi pamphlets to other Germans, they were paying the ultimate price of death for their ideals and for their attempt to save the lives of others. As they died most of these students, who previously had experienced a great love of life, now felt that their individual death had value and was in God's timing.

One young man Christoph Probst wrote to his mother (in a letter which she never received but was only allowed to see briefly):

> I thank you that you gave me life. When I think about it, it was the only way to God. Don't be sad that I sprang over part of it. Soon I'll be much closer to you than ever, I'll prepare all of you a glorious reception. . . .[10]

If, however, it is a principle of Scripture that human life is of high value, it is also a principle that *life* is to be prolonged, not the dying process. Our living and our dying are to be in God's time, with our dying neither prolonged nor cut short.

Defining the Moment of Death

Just as we feel the need to define *life* in terms that speak to modern technology, so also one might ask, "What is *death*?" Death used to be obvious. When a person ceased to respond to life and stopped breathing, they were dead, or soon would be, because nothing more could be done. Today machines have an escalating capacity to keep the human body "alive."

The generally referred to standard for determining death is still that formulated by the Ad Hoc Committee of the Harvard Medical School in 1968. This definition requires total brain death. More specifically, it cites four main criteria:

1. Unreceptivity and unresponsivity
2. No movements or breathing
3. No reflexes
4. Flat electroencephalogram[11]

When artificial means are available to prolong life, further definition of death may be required. In 1972 it was proposed that:

> In the event that artificial means of support preclude a determination that these functions have ceased, a person will be considered dead if in the announced opinion of a physician, based on ordinary standards of medical practice, he has experienced an irreversible cessation of spontaneous brain function.[12]

Defining death is no longer a simple matter. If a person dies in a remote area where help will not be available for hours, the determination of death will be rather clear-cut. They will simply not respond and, eventually, there will be all sorts of evidence of death. But in cases where the help of medical technology *is* available, it will probably not be that easy. It is sometimes difficult to draw the line between treating life and prolonging dying or even treating a dead corpse.

Billy Graham cites the view of death expressed by Edith Schaeffer, wife of the late Francis Schaeffer:

> For years she and Francis had talked about the preciousness of life and that even a few minutes could make a difference if something needed to be said or done. "But," she said, "there is no point in simply prolonging death. It is a fine line; it is not an absolute one-two-three process. There are differences from person to person, and it requires great wisdom."[13]

For with all our new technologies, the precise moment at which a person is truly dead is not always so easy to define. Comments Richard G. Benton in *Death and Dying*: "As the situation now stands, a person may be considered alive in one hospital and considered dead according to another definition employed in a hospital across town."[14] Moreover, from a very technical point of view, "Individuals who are apparently destroyed in a sudden manner, by certain wounds, diseases or even decapitation, are not really dead, but are only in a condition incompatible with the persistence of life."[15] Explains Benton; "Any youngster on a farm could confirm that observation—chop off a chicken's head and the body will run around wildly without the head."[16]

In essence, death does not come immediately. When I was watching my Aunt Lydia as she was dying, it reminded me of the computer which I had just bought: she seemed to shut down, system by system. Death was a process. And the slower the process, the harder it is to know when a person is truly dying and cannot be brought back to life, or when intervention will in fact prolong life.

There are attempts being made to redefine death away from the current standard of total brain death. Some of these attempts arise from a desire to clarify that which is so confusing. Others of these efforts have been attempts to clarify the point at which organs may be taken for transplants. Still other such attempts, as in the case of anencephalic infants, have been related to attempts to declare certain human beings non-human so that their tissues and organs can be used freely for transplantations and experimentation.

Some now believe that when the outer part of the brain, the cerebral cortex, which is responsible for the more complicated human functions like thinking, dies, death has occurred, even though the brain stem, which controls physical processes, remains alive. Thus, they reason, when cerebral death occurs a respirator can be turned off.

I am not at all sure that one must wait for death, by whatever definition, in order to turn off a respirator. If one is treating life, then to stop treatment would be to kill. However, if one is merely prolonging the dying process, after what may have been a valid attempt to save that life which is now obviously dying, then I see no reason to keep machines going.

However, I have a problem with using *cerebral* death as a definition of death because this reinforces our current overemphasis on intellectual ability as a basis for worth. It also sets an arbitrary, man-made standard for death which has to ignore the obvious fact that something is still going on in this person, even if I as a human being don't consider that "something" to be of value.

There are other moral issues which relate to the use of cerebral death as an overall definition of death: once again, the concepts of *life unworthy of life* or *quality of life* become an issue. Anencephalic babies who are born with little or no cerebral cortex would have to logically be declared non-human if the presence of a live-cerebral-cortex definition of life. Thus one category of being whom God has made would be disqualified from being in God's image.

Maybe God has given us these babies and others, who may have cerebral function but would still be considered "defective" in intelligence, to show us that cerebral function is not the only value which God puts on a human being. I am reminded again of the friend who was so impressed by the loving dispositions of the Down's Syndrome children he worked with. If, in God's sight, all of our works are *nothing* without love, we should think twice about considering any intellectually "defective" person non-human.

And again, if cerebral death were the standard, these anencephalic babies and anyone else whose brain stem remained alive after cerebral death would be fair game for transplantation and experimentation. Such a position is just one step closer to the day when organs are "farmed" (as seen in the movie *Coma*). Pretty soon those with Alzheimer's, the severely retarded, certainly the unborn, and others would become open prey. Let us never forget that in Germany euthanasia started with the terminally ill and those in chronic pain and ended up with killing those with misshapen ear lobes and bed wetters!

Three Helpful Principles From the Bible

Volumes could be written on all the what-ifs of medical technology. But we are on much safer ground if we follow certain general biblical principles . . . whether or not we like them. For otherwise we are in desperate danger of trying to become gods and making our own rules based on what we feel and what we want at any given moment. Basically those biblical principles can be summarized in three statements: the sanctity of all human life; the sovereignty of God, including his timing in matters of life and death; and the goodness of God, who will not fail to do right.

We get into trouble when we question any of these principles. Questions like: "What would Aunt Sally want?" are not designed to find out the will of God in bioethics. They merely express what we want or feel. "What is the will of God?" is a more appropriate question for the believer. Fundamental to the Judeo-Christian tradition is an absolute reliance on the will of God.

It is a violation of the sanctity of life to *keep* a person here on earth *beyond* God's timing, just as it is to take that same person too soon. This thought was evidently in the late Joe Bayly's mind when he faced death and wrote:

Lord
if anything happens
if you come for me
keep them from interfering
desperately trying
to tug me
from your grasp.
If I'm far
across the river
where you own the shore
and all beyond
don't let them
bring me back
prolonging death
not life
delaying life
that never crosses
the unreturning river
again.[17]

For the Christian death is not an end; it is a transition into eternal reward. The end is not scary, but the process can be. Certainly that process should not be prolonged or shortened, for each moment which God has for a human being on this earth is planned from throughout all eternity. And each moment spent in heaven is planned with equal precision. We don't want to be here, when we should be there; nor do we want to be there, when God still wants us here. This earth has a purpose, to prepare us for heaven. And only God holds that timing in his hand.

It takes great godliness not to go to extremes. In my counseling office I hear good Christians talk about going to great extremes to prolong the dying process while others seem ready to go for euthanasia, based, not on the will of God, but on how they feel. When we base such decisions on our own desires or logic rather than on biblical principles, we can easily fall into error.

As Christians who value God's gift of life we do not have the right to refuse treatment where treatment can restore us to life, even if that treatment is painful or if we are too depressed to want it. Nor, conversely, are we obligated to bring someone back from death when it is clear that we cannot bring them back to life but only to dying once again in the immediate future.

In terms of actual practice, there is a frighteningly direct relationship between the issue of how far to treat and euthanasia. If we glorify the dying process and the value of pain, and if we force people to think that sanctity of life means going to ridiculous and tormenting extremes, many will give up altogether and opt for the easiest way out—assisted suicide or euthanasia. Legalism can produce an abandonment of principle in that it makes principle appear to be unattainable. Harshness in the place of love can deter people from God rather than draw them to him. It is possible to deter people from a good cause by using extreme methods. Let us remember that moderation, as well as sanctity of life, is a principle of Scripture (Philippians 4:5).

There are grey areas, however, and in these areas in particular we are required by God to love and support those that make decisions which differ from ours. We will not always agree. A respirator, for example, is a very uncomfortable piece of equipment to be attached to; and its use is still a matter of controversy among doctors. The prospect of being on a respirator is one of my own greatest personal fears, along with paralysis and stroke. Consequently I have great sympathy for those who arbitrarily let it be known that under no conditions do they wish to be put on this machine, even to save their lives. If that respirator can be a bridge back to life, however, we have an obligation to try to live. If, on the other hand, the respirator is used when death is inevitable, simply to slow the dying process, then that is wrongfully keeping a person from being released to be with God.

Referring to the Karen Quinlan case, in which there was debate over the ethics of turning off life-support machines, the editors of *Law and Bioethics* commented:

> We glean from the record here that physicians distinguish between curing the ill and comforting and easing the dying; that they refuse to treat the curable as if they were dying or ought to die, and that they have sometimes refused to treat the hopeless and dying as if they were curable.[18]

In his statement relating to the same case, Pope Pius XII made the point that:

> This case is not to be considered euthanasia in any way; that would never be licit. The interruption of attempts at resuscitation, even when it causes the arrest of circulation, is not more than an indirect cause of the cessation of life.[19]

Death Should Be a Time of Dignity

Too many deaths today are needlessly torturous. It is important for the medical profession to get back to the art of comforting the dying and supplying whatever is needed in personal contact as well as drugs, oxygen, fluids, and even nutrients which make death an easier death. For as we have seen, "easy death" was the original meaning of the term euthanasia! It has only in relatively recent times come to mean killing. Those last moments on earth can be very important ones for each of us as we go to face our Maker. For some it is the place of decision. For others it becomes a point of loving transition. And for the family, rather than the deathbed being a frantic place, it can be a place of blessing from the one who is so close to being at home with his Lord.

In a recent issue of *Decision* John White says:

> In life we are on a stage. Angels and demons watch as we enact the drama of our earthly existence, and it is important that the scene close properly. Christ has shown us how the lines should

be uttered, as a cry of joyful triumph: "Father, into thy hands I commit my spirit!" [Luke 23:46, RSV] We will only die once and will therefore have only one chance to die properly. We must learn our lines well beforehand so that the curtains fall on a note of triumph.[20]

It has been obvious from the outset of our discussion on euthanasia and how far to treat that the boundaries are blurred, at times, between active euthanasia, passive euthanasia, and natural death. The term passive euthanasia can be a very confusing one and is often used as an argument *for* euthanasia. Those who do this point out that everything from outright refusal of valid treatment down to over-eating and smoking are passive euthanasia. Therefore, according to these people, you might just a well believe in euthanasia since you can't help but live by it the first time you neglect some aspect of health care. To me such an argument is purposefully deceptive and ultimately ridiculous. It makes all of us who live in California smog purposefully, if ever so slowly, suicidal! However, to know when we are not treating enough and thus are in danger of performing *real* passive euthanasia is perhaps the most difficult question for those of us who firmly believe in the sanctity of life.

How far to treat is an issue which generates great confusion for many. I once met someone who claimed that his brain waves were flat after an accident and that the doctors gave him up. He was kept on machines at the insistence of his family, well after normal medical criteria would have declared him dead. Yet several days later he came back to consciousness with seemingly no brain damage. It would probably be impossible for this man to ever feel right in turning off a respirator without total brain death as a prerequisite. "Severe barbiturate poisoning has also produced cases of flat EEG readings in which the patients recovered." Yet the presence of flat EEG's has long been a standard in determining death.[21]

A similar case involved a Norwegian youngster who was nearly drowned, having been submerged in a freezing river for twenty-two minutes. After touch-and-go emergency measures such as heart massage, drug injections, and blood transfusions, his vital functions started to work spontaneously. Later, "he relapsed into total unconsciousness for five weeks and during part of this time had no measurable brain function at all: in the jargon he was "decerebrate." However ... six months later he was back at home, a normal child again.[22]

Most of us can tell stories of seemingly miraculous recoveries. Some are unexplainable except by the intervention of God himself. Others are probably just inaccurate, either in the recounting or in the actual perception of the medical potential at that time. Future research may offer some explanation. In the interim, such incidents cannot be disregarded, and they should, indeed, slow us down in giving up on life too quickly. However, they cannot totally influence us in our decision making, since they remain still the exception rather than the rule.

Defining "Extraordinary" Treatment

There are other issues of how far to treat, apart from definitions of death and the use of respirators to sustain life. Forced feeding is in the forefront of these issues: some regard it as extraordinary treatment, while to others it is minimal care. Perhaps here, as in so many issues, the *motive* should be the determining factor. If a baby survives an abortion and is left in the room to starve to death, or if a seriously defective baby born full term is left neglected in a room to die, that is killing. On the other hand, forced feeding in order to prolong the dying process seems inappropriate *unless* it is done in order to make the patient more comfortable. For example, when my Aunt Lydia was dying she became restless and dehydrated. Fluids were given intravenously in order to soothe the dying process, not to prolong it.

It is dangerous, in my opinion, to set up rigid rules regarding treatment. For example, stopping dialysis arbitrarily at age fifty-five puts a value judgment on how much a given person can benefit from treatment, based on his age alone; and it judges a person's worth on the same standard.

To stop dialysis because of a well thought out decision is another issue altogether. A young man who had cancer entered the terminal state where chemotherapy caused great discomfort and accomplished less and less. At the same time he was receiving dialysis. The day came when he discontinued both treatments because he was in great pain and knew that he would die very soon in any case. I personally do not feel that his decision was wrong.

The rationing of medical services is talked about a great deal today, as we saw in chapter 1. There are, however, inherent dangers in such thinking. To say arbitrarily that a certain number of treatments will be allowed each person for a given disease, based on usual amounts needed, is to risk improper treatment for some who, with a little extra treatment, might go on living. In *The New England Journal of Medicine* in 1973, Dr. Leo Alexander commented wisely on a situation where electroconvulsive treatments per patient were limited to thirty-five per year:

> Two years ago if a physician performed an abortion he was a criminal, but if subsequently, after his patient went into a severe depression, he brought about her recovery by 48 electroconvulsive treatments, he was a good doctor. Now the situation is reversed: when he performs the abortion he is a good doctor, but if he subsequently finds it necessary to relieve her severe depression by 40 electroconvulsive treatments, he will be a criminal. Such laws, in comparison to our Hippocratic obligation, enduring throughout the entire history of medicine, are merely words written into sand.[23]

So, it would seem today, may be the fate of the Hippocratic Oath. It too may prove to have been written in sand, thereby endangering the consistency of patient care for all who need it.

As we approach the end of the twentieth century, medicine is becoming focused on interesting experiments rather than on routine patient care. We are starting to limit patient treatment by economic restrictions. Many people do not qualify for good medical insurance while others cannot afford it. General health care is in a state of chaos in spite of state-of-the-art technology. The result is once again a diminishing of the value of human life.

During the Nuremberg trials of Nazi war criminals, the accusations became so bizarre that Judge Parker, unable to accept the extremes of horror, returned to his house one night and said to his aide: "You know, Jim, they're going too far in this trial. They claimed today that the guards threw babies up and shot them in the camps. You know no one would do that."

Not long after this exchange Judge Parker and the others saw a short forty-five minute film:

Its images stayed with anyone who saw it. It showed the warehouse at Maidanek where 800,000 pairs of shoes had been neatly stacked, the piles of skulls, broken bodies, mutilated corpses. There were sequences where naked women were driven to mass graves; they lay down and were shot; the guards smiled for the camera.

The film was the most horrifying evidence which had been introduced. Judge Parker went to bed for three days after viewing it. Even the defendants reacted with shock. Only Hitler's henchman Goering seemed bored, yawned at appropriate moments and read a book.[24]

At the end of the trial, with the defendants convicted, many of them with the death sentence, there was a small but significant example of how deeply a sense of the sanctity of life was instilled into those who were part of that court at Nuremberg. At other times there had been celebrations when their work was over:

Tonight there was little celebration. Most people felt depressed and went home quietly to pack. It is a terrible thing to see a man condemned to death even when you are certain that he has been responsible for the death of millions.[25]

When all was said and done, even the life of a Nazi killer could only be terminated with sadness. Such is the meaning of the sanctity of life.

NINE

Question Marks

It was a late Sunday afternoon. It was fall, but the sun was bright and the air was balmy and warm. Four children, each of whom had been a victim of abuse, and a friend and I were spending the afternoon walking along the beach, picking up shells, and idly throwing rocks back into the sea. As the afternoon turned into evening, and the sun began to set over the ocean, we sat down in the sand and quietly watched its magnificence.

"My mother died last winter," one boy, Jon, said, breaking into the stillness. "My Dad used to beat her," he added slowly. "Is she in heaven?"

Before I could answer his question his eight-year-old friend asked, "Where's heaven? Is it up in the sky above that sunset?"

Another child, looking at me with a penetrating perception beyond her six years, asked: "Are your parents still alive?"

When I replied "No," she asked me where they were. "In heaven," I answered quietly.

"Can they see us at this very minute?" she continued. "Do you think they know what we are doing?"

Jon quickly added, "If my mom is there, do you think they know each other?"

The fourth child, a ten-year-old boy, spoke for the first

time. "Let's talk," he suggested. "Sometimes when my Dad used to get drunk and I was home with him alone, I would remember a story I heard in Sunday school about angels. It helped me to think that angels were going to protect me from my Dad. What are angels, anyway?"

So we talked, till long after the sun had dropped like a large, fiery ball into the sea. We talked about God and angels and heaven. We talked about many of the question marks which man has always had about that unseen world around us. Above all, we talked about how each of them could come to know God by accepting Christ as their personal Lord and Savior. To do so would not mean the eradication of pain in their lives, nor would it mean that they would never have unanswered questions. But, if they came to know Christ, the biggest question mark of all would be answered. They would never again have to question their eternal destiny. One thing which does not need to be a question mark is our salvation. God never changes!

The late Alfred J. Crick, that dear Plymouth Brethren Bible teacher from England, described conversion as "the moment when I decided that God's will must be mine and I slipped into that wonderful sphere."[1] Since that day on the beach, several of those children have made a commitment to Jesus Christ and have "slipped into that wonderful sphere" of a personal walk with God which will last throughout all eternity.

For a moment on that beach my mind drifted off to the issues which have been addressed in this book, and it occurred to me that with all of the technological advances of the twentieth century, as we enter the twenty-first century we have more questions than ever. Moreover, for every answer given there have been just that many more questions created.

Then, as my thoughts went back to my conversation with these children who knew so little of God, I realized anew that the only answers which haven't changed are those which relate to God himself. In a changing world, he alone is unchangeable.

Avoiding the Truth

Sometimes in life we not only do not know the answers to certain questions, but we do not even want to deal with the issues involved. Truth is too painful, so we avoid it. Since the Holocaust there has been much criticism against a world which did so little to help rescue the Jewish people. Evidence of indifference and anti-Semitism cannot be ignored. But among many people, Jewish and non-Jewish alike, there was also a tendency to avoid the truth, to dismiss reliable reports as too horrible to be believed.

During the summer of 1942, a report was smuggled out from Poland. It told of the mass-gassing of 700,000 Jews at Chelmno. In detail the report described how the victims were told to undress for a bath. Then they were directed down a hallway and forced into an open truck. The truck was driven to a deep ditch in a nearby woods, where the truck itself became a gas chamber. Jewish gravediggers were forced to unload the bodies, and German workers stripped them of all gold teeth and jewelry. Then they were buried in layers in the ditch. This process of killing was repeated several times. Eventually most of the gravediggers were also killed.

Three of the gravediggers escaped to tell the story to the Jewish underground. Yet American mass media did not mention the story, nor did most of the Jewish press . . . "apparently because the story seemed so incredible." As the editor of one Jewish publication said a quarter of a century later: "Such things did not happen in the twentieth century."[2]

A year earlier, in 1941, a man they called Moshe the Beadle lived in a little town in Transylvania. He was poor and humble, but he had great knowledge. A twelve-year-old boy, Elie Wiesel, also lived in the village. The twelve-year-old was told that he was too young to engage in certain studies. So he found his own teacher in Moshe the Beadle. The two spent hours talking.

Moshe explained to the boy that, "Man raises himself

toward God by the questions he asks him."

Then the day came when all foreign Jews were ordered to leave the village. Moshe the Beadle was a foreigner.

Eventually Moshe returned. But he had changed and his joy was gone. He told his story:

> The train full of deportees had crossed the Hungarian frontier and on Polish territory had been taken in charge by the Gestapo. There it had stopped. The Jews had to climb out and climb into lorries. The lorries drove toward a forest. The Jews were made to get out. They were made to dig huge graves. And when they had finished their work, the Gestapo began theirs. Without passion, without haste, they slaughtered their prisoners. Each one had to go up to the hole and present his neck. Babies were thrown into the air and the machine gunners used them as targets.[3]

Moshe had been left for dead. But in truth he had only been wounded. So he escaped and told his story, from one house to another. But no one would believe him. It was too fantastic to believe. In the town where Elie Wiesel was growing up they didn't believe the story either. Life went on. Hope persisted. It was now spring of 1944.

Then the soldiers came, and it was too late for the Jews to believe what they had heard. Now even Moshe the Beadle was silent, except for the words: "I warned you. . . ."[4]

We Must Heed the Warning Signs

At this time in our history we are at a point where medical technology can replace heart valves and, in many other ways, extend a life by years. We can shrink a cancerous growth with radiation. We can perform a multitude of tests which graphically show the most intricate workings of almost every part of the human body. We can do surgery on an unborn baby while it is still in the womb. With the use of the laser we can perform surgery without ever making an incision. Medical "miracles" have become routine. Yet this progress has not come about without its corresponding nightmare, which calls for a warning as strong and as uncompromising as the one brought by Moshe the Beadle.

In September of 1988 a pill called RU-486 was put on the market in France, where it was developed. In essence the pill prevents the fertilized egg, the zygote, from attaching itself to the uterine wall, thus causing it to abort itself. This particular pill is effective only during the first seven weeks of pregnancy, and usually it is taken within three weeks after a woman's first missed menstrual cycle. RU-486, or any pill like it, provides the option of a private abortion without anyone's knowledge, including the father! Some even suggest that it be taken routinely, without even the mother's knowledge of pregnancy. In that way no sense of responsibility need be experienced! I consider this to be abortion, not contraception.

In April 1989, *Los Angeles Times Magazine* reported on a *too successful* attempt at in vitro fertilization. A woman flown in from a small midwestern town had tried unsuccessfully to conceive, . . .

> but in recent weeks, after in vitro fertilization, she had five embryos implanted in her womb and all five unexpectedly began to thrive. Now, the odds are not in her favor for a healthy pregnancy unless he (the doctor) uses his technical mastery: He must end the lives of three fetuses. Kill three to save two.

Commented one doctor: "We've got some doctors putting in extra babies only to turn to another doctor and ask him to get rid of a couple of them" . . . or, in this case, three of them![5]

Two middle aged couples sat talking together over a late supper in a restaurant overlooking downtown Los Angeles. One of the ladies commented: "One of our friends died last month, and the wonderful part was that until the end she could think clearly. I hope when I die I'm like that. Not being able to think clearly and remember is what frightens me about ever having Alzheimer's."

Her husband started to agree with her, when his business partner sitting across from him interrupted with enthusiasm: "Haven't you heard?" he asked. "These days they can take fetal tissue . . . you know from the unborn in abortions . . . and transplant the tissue into those who have Alzheimer's. That way the tissue doesn't get rejected when it replaces the diseased tissue."

There was an awkward silence as the first couple attempted to absorb this new piece of medical technology. Then they changed the subject. But they remembered enough to bring it up to me when I saw them next. They were somewhat horrified, but they were also intrigued with such potential. They might not approve now, but perhaps in the near future, if they were in need. . . .

It is becoming easy in our world to begin to ignore the principle of the sanctity of life when it affects *us*. When *my* daughter wants an abortion. . . . When I want euthanasia because it meets *my* needs. . . . When I don't want to endure a painful treatment which can prolong my life. . . . Life and death are becoming choices we think we can make on our own, rather than being under the authority of God. Body parts and tissue transplants are close to becoming commercial commodities to barter and sell. We, like the villagers who were warned by Moshe the Beadle, tend to ignore the warnings which are increasingly all around us. Will we, like them, wait until it is too late?

The late U.S. senator Hubert Humphrey said: "The ethical test of a society is how it treats those who are in the dawn of life, the children, those who are in the twilight of life, the aged, and those who are in the shadows of life, the sick and the needy."[6] These are the people who are in danger from today's confusion about medical ethics combined with the escalating price of health care. These will be the experimented upon, the abused, the used, and the ignored.

But the rest of us are not exempt. No one was exempt in the Third Reich. Hitler himself died violently, by his own hand, as the nightmarish empire he had created began to fall apart.

A woman who survived the sinking of the *Titanic* said that originally her family had been scheduled to sail on a different vessel, and her mother was experiencing great anxiety about the perils of sea travel. Then, by seeming coincidence, the family was transferred to the *Titanic*, that huge traveling palace with its lavish staterooms. The *Titanic* was called unsinkable, and carried on its fatal maiden voyage the rich and famous of the world. This particular family's friends envied their luck in being able to travel on the maiden voyage of that great vessel. The mother's anxiety increased, however, rather than subsiding. When her husband tried to reassure her with the fact that everyone was calling the *Titanic* unsinkable, she replied that it was the very fact which frightened her: it was as if they were going in the face of God.

Just as the Tower of Babel in the Old Testament defied the authority and power of God, so in our quest to take over the control of our own medical destiny we are in danger of going in the face of God. If we wait until death becomes mandatory at seventy; or dialysis is refused at fifty-five; or death is mandated for Alzheimer's or mental retardation or AIDS; if we wait until there are mandatory abortions for the poor or the "genetically unsound," whoever they may be; if we wait until organs are taken from live bodies which are warehoused in a perfectly controlled environment; if we wait until others tell us what we may do with our own bodies . . . we will have waited too long for anything but the collapse of our entire society to save us.

Those who promote voluntary euthanasia don't tell us that historically voluntary euthanasia has always turned into *involuntary* euthanasia. They don't explain that many individuals who promote abortion also support the infanticide of the "unfit," or mandatory abortion in certain instances, or a return to forced sterilization. As some said back in the forties, it takes long preparation to get a society to condone such acts, and so we only hear of these things gradually, one by one, starting with those issues which will gain the easiest support.

It has been a common argument of those who promote voluntary euthanasia, for example, to urge the need for an "easy" death. They talk about terminal illness and chronic pain. Yet most authorities on euthanasia, even those in the Netherlands, admit that pain is low on the list of reasons for requests for euthanasia. In the same way, while pro-abortionists talk about incest, rape, and danger to a woman's life, comparatively few people who want abortions want them for those reasons. But it is easier to convince people of the validity of euthanasia if you talk about chronic pain; and it is easier to convince someone of the validity of abortion if you talk about rape. Then, from chronic pain and rape, it is easy to begin to add other reasons which sound valid. That is, indeed, the opening of Pandora's box. And even for Pandora, once the box was opened it could not be closed.

An eyewitness to an accident on a California freeway described it as follows:

> The red car was following a large truck in the far left lane. Then the red car turned right into the next lane. In a few seconds the truck also moved right into the next lane. Again, the red car moved right and then the truck moved right, still in front of the red car by two car lengths. Still again the woman in the red car moved right, this time into the far right lane, beyond which there was only a broken fence and some thick growth of bushes and weeds. For the last time, the right turn signal lights went on at the rear end of the truck as the driver began to edge into the far right lane, still well ahead of the red car.

"Then," said the witness, "I saw the lady in the red car throw up her hands and head her car toward the bushes! She just threw up her hands and headed for the bushes!"

In the area of medical ethics and technology, many today are not even thinking long-range. Many of us who do see some of the long-range issues prefer to postpone facing them. Others who see have already given up and just feel that there are no real answers. For whatever our reasons, we as a society are throwing up our hands and heading for the bushes at a time when clear thinking and godly perception are more needed than ever before.

Lighthouses

Last winter I spent a long weekend by the ocean. It was one of those times of ideal, refurbishing retreat which occur infrequently in most of our lives. Combining good friends, a small but meaningful worship service on the Lord's Day, and the backdrop of a rugged, scenic coastline, the weekend provided a safety zone in the middle of heavy demands. The peak of enjoyment for me was an unexpected afternoon spent at the old Point Loma lighthouse. Going there was a spur-of-the-moment decision based only on the fact that none of us had ever been there before.

The view from the lighthouse has been judged to be one of the three greatest harbor views in the world, an opinion which seemed justified to me that afternoon even before I read it later in a book. On the day of our visit, the fog was thick and the wind brisk. As I walked up the rather steep hill to the lighthouse I had a sense of peaceful exhilaration. Then as the lighthouse itself came into full view, there seemed to be so many spiritual applications. There it was, high above the earth on a hill with one sole function: to throw light into the darkness in order to warn ships of the rocky coast below and to direct them to safety.

I thought of John 1:4-5,9 where it says of Christ:

In Him was Life, and that Life was the Light of men. The Light shines in the darkness, and darkness has not overpowered it. . . . The true Light was that which illumines every man by its coming into the world (Weymouth).

Then I remembered a verse which is a sort of counterpart to that verse:

You are the light of the world. A town [or, a lighthouse] on the top of a hill cannot be hidden. Nor do men light a lamp to put it under a bowl; they put it on a stand, and it shines for all in the house. So your light is to shine before men, that they may see the good you do and glorify your Father in heaven (Matthew 5:14-16, Moffatt).

I learned that the responsibility of the keeper of this lighthouse had always been to have the lighting equipment in good order by ten in the morning so that there would be no chance that the light would not shine each night. Wicks were trimmed, lenses cleaned and polished, for otherwise the light produced by the whale oil would not show through. All this had to be accomplished by the beginning of the day, not in a hurry right before its use was required.

What a picture this portrays of the life of the individual Christian: cleansed of sin, filled with the Spirit, prepared daily, and shedding a light into the darkness of the world around—a light which not only warns of danger but directs to safety.

An interesting fact which is unique to the Point Loma lighthouse is that it was built high on top of a hill in order to more effectively cast its light over the sea below. But then it was discovered that, because it was so high above the earth, sometimes the fog rolled in between the ocean and the lighthouse rather than above it, and the light would become obscured.

It has been said that as Christians we can be so high above the earth that we are no earthly good. I have always disliked that statement, for it seems to imply that too much godliness diminishes our ability to serve God. The opposite is true. The more we live in the heavenlies, so to speak, the more we will be able to serve God on this earth. We cannot live too closely to God. However there is a tendency in many Christians to disconnect ourselves from the practical problems of this earth. We don't like to see the unpleasant. Some who started this book will never read these words, because some of the previous chapters will have been too unpleasant, too disturbing. These people will be like the lighthouse, equipped to manifest that Light of the World, Jesus Christ himself, but unwilling to come off the mountain and see through the fog and view the unpleasantness of those shipwrecked on the rocks below.

It is impossible to make changes in this world and to act in love toward those in need if we stay in our safe little neighborhoods and never see real, live human beings who are hurting. It is impossible to have opinions about the warehousing of body parts, if we've never heard of it. It is impossible to vote intelligently about voluntary euthanasia when it appears on our ballot, as it has already in some states, if we've never thought about it before and if we do not understand its long-range potential.

A friend of mine often remarks about a "bag lady" whom she encounters, it seems, almost every time she goes grocery shopping or anywhere else around town. The sight of this lady always disturbed my friend, but up to a week ago that was as far as it went. Then last week she dropped by my apartment after work and enthusiastically said: "I saw the bag lady again." Not perceiving anything of particular interest in her statement, since she always seemed to see her, I made some casual comment in response.

"You don't understand," she continued. "I decided I couldn't just go by and pretend she wasn't there. So I went over to McDonald's and bought a cheeseburger, some fries, and a carton of milk. Then I went back and gave them to her. I found out her name and we talked."

Now, thoroughly interested, I asked, "What did she say?"

"Not much," my friend said. "But she seemed surprised when I asked her name. And as I left I looked back, and I noticed that she was no longer hunched up, looking down at the sidewalk. She had picked her sweater up off the sidewalk where people could walk on it, and she was sipping her milk."

The light from the lighthouse had reached the earth and had penetrated one small piece of the darkness.

One Small Light

Sometimes we feel that because we are a minority of one we can't do much. One small light doesn't seem to light up the darkness very much. A young man went to the market and included in his groceries a box of matzos. As the box boy was putting his groceries into a bag, he exclaimed with contempt, "This is Jewish food." The man was upset enough to decide never to shop in that store again, but he felt too intimidated to say anything. "I just wanted to run," he said later.

That evening, however, he could not get the incident out of his mind. What was really troubling him was the fact that he had remained silent. In a moment of decision he pick up the telephone, called the store, and asked for the manager. The result was immediate: an apology from the box boy! And certainly at least one market is a little more aware that they can't get by with even small actions of anti-Semitism. The light penetrated the darkness.

Throughout the history of mankind it has been proven that one man can make a difference. Biblical history alone is filled with powerful examples. In Genesis 19:29 we read that "God remembered Abraham" and therefore saved Lot and his family. Queen Esther—one young woman—convinced the king to save God's people of Israel during her lifetime. Likewise Moses, one man, led the entire Jewish nation out of their life of slavery in Egypt.

Closer to our own day, one of the people to whom this book is dedicated, Raoul Wallenberg, was responsible for the saving of 100,000 Jews in Budapest at the end of World War II during only a nine month period. He performed remarkable acts of courage as he literally ordered people out of the cattle cars which were to transport them to the concentration camps and at the same moment threatened the Gestapo with punishment from their own leaders if they opposed him! Since then he has languished in Soviet prison camps, forgotten for most of those years by a world which wanted to forget.

The magnitude of Wallenberg's courage is only emphasized by the reasons which have been given for his arrest. It has been assumed by some that he had to be a spy, for otherwise why would the wealthy son of a banking family from a neutral country like Sweden get involved in saving Jews? As one officer said at the time, with a roar of laughter: "Do you really think that any sensible person would believe that people would stay in this town under siege, just for 'humanitarian purposes' when they could have returned to their nice peaceful neutral country!"[7]

Some today would declare: "Raoul Wallenberg was an unusual man. He was brave. I am not brave. I cannot perform such acts of bravery." Yet according to biographer Kati Marton:

> The courage of Wallenberg displayed that fall and winter of 1944 was all the more startling because it was not based on a natural fearlessness. More than anything else, Wallenberg's bravery was a product of will. The calm he exhibited in the most unnerving situations did not come easily to him. He was not by nature a man who embraced brinkmanship.... He was very young and had a healthy appetite for life.[8]

He was one man who chose to become extraordinary!

The man who was with him at that time and shared in many of the risks as well as the triumphs is also included in this dedication. For during just one speech and one interview, Swedish Ambassador Per Anger imprinted upon my emotions, more than perhaps any other person, the potential for influence which exists within one human being.

In a telling footnote in his book on Wallenberg, biographer John Bierman wrote of Ambassador Anger:

> With characteristic modesty, Anger failed to mention that he made some forays to the border without Wallenberg and was personally responsible for a number of rescues. In 1956, when he was attached to the Swedish embassy in Vienna, he again went to the Austro-Hungarian border to help refugees from the Soviet takeover that followed the Budapest uprising of that year. He told the author how he saw a group of people coming across the border, including some Jewish women, one of whom fell into his arms and said: "Per Anger, this is the second time you have saved me."[9]

Another example, from that same era, of individual courage involved a Catholic bishop:

> In 1941 a Catholic biship, Clemens August (Count von) Galen could bear no more. He had long been a critic of the Nazis, and as far back as 1934 he had spoken out against their racial policies. That July, in 1941, he stood up in his church and thundered his outrage at a program that was "against God's commandments, against the law of nature, and against the system of jurisprudence of Germany." He roared at his congregation, "These are our brothers and sisters!" and asked them how they expected to live if the measure of their life span was economic productivity. No one's life was safe any longer, he said, and he then asked who now could have confidence in his doctor.[10]

Galen's sermon circulated all over Germany, appearing in the mailboxes of Protestants as well as Catholics. Once again, as in the case of Raoul Wallenberg, one man made a difference.

In the Christian, the potential for what one man or woman can do is at its peak, for we go, not in our own power, but in the power of God himself. We have, indeed, an obligation to act. In the words of that Gentile martyr of the Holocaust, Lutheran pastor Dietrich Bonhoeffer, as he wrote from his prison cell, "Mere waiting and looking on is not Christian behaviour."[11]

Light . . . and Darkness

As we approach the twenty-first century and deal with the confusion and tragedies of our own times, the principles remain the same. God remains the same. The choice to act in wisdom and in love is ever present as an option and as an obligation. There will be times when the fog will roll in beneath us, and we will not always see with clarity.

Even within the medical profession itself there is often a great ignorance and confusion regarding medical ethics. As I have talked informally with various physicians, remarks have been dropped which are alarming. Some have not seemed to know that under Roe v. Wade abortion could be available through nine months of pregnancy. Others are more concerned about their legal protection than they are about the protection of human lives. As one physician said: "When the patient is in a coma on a respirator, I don't worry about the patient. I worry about the family. The patient will probably die, but the family will be alive and able to sue!"

Some physicians were more blunt than others. Many of these physicians are well trained, likeable, and effective, but in my opinion have looked at the issues, thrown up their hands and "headed for the bushes." The problems of too much technology, too many sick people, too little in the way of financial resources, and a society which wants everyone to have everything but does not want to pay for it, overwhelm many in the medical community. These men are good doctors, but they are trained in medicine, not in social welfare or economics. Many of them are simply waiting for direction from a society which is also floundering in the confusion of current medical issues.

Those who believe that man is truly made in the image of God have an obligation to clarify and promote a view of man which says a resounding no to medicalized killing for *any* reason. Such a view of God does not allow for dehumanizing euphemisms like "product of conception," which places the unborn outside the realm of legal protection. Nor does it support the tolerance of pre-Holocaust Germans when their courts declared Jewish people to be non-human, thereby placing them, too, outside the protection of the law. Unless we clarify our views on these matters, and make those views known, we will drift in a sea of misguided medical ethics . . . until those ethics affect us personally. And then it may be too late.

Meanwhile, the confusion just deepens as medical technology increases, and finances often determine the extent and quality of medical care. Based on the widespread premise that not everyone can get adequate treatment, Dr. Ian Jones, head of obstetrics and gynecology at Scripps Clinic in La Jolla, California, stated the feelings and asked the questions of many doctors: "Society has to decide whether it wants to kill things; and if it does, well then kill them, but don't erect this huge kind of ethical dilemma about it to which there is no solution." Continuing, he explained: "I'd just as soon society would decide whether it wants to kill people or doesn't. If it does, well, that's fine; and if it doesn't, that's fine too."

In talking about how one adjusts to such killing, Dr. Jones continued, using the example of the slaughterhouse. You couldn't eat meat if "every time you ate a piece of steak you thought of this warm calf with its wet nose that had just been feeding from its mother a half hour before, then some ugly man in the slaughterhouse went 'bang' and killed it. . . . I think it's the same thing with euthanasia and abortion."

In formulating his views on medical ethics, Dr. Jones does not deny the reality of life in the womb. With rhetoric which was refreshingly free from euphemisms in speaking of the unborn, Dr. Jones asked: "Does it really matter when a fetus is a child?" Then, answering his own question: "No. I mean, a baby is a baby whether it's in or out of the uterus. The only difference is it hasn't been born yet. That's all."

Yet in talking of the growing demands on medical care, Dr. Jones expressed an opinion I have heard from others who feel that there is an inevitable conflict between the idealism of unlimited health care services and the problems of supply and demand:

> When there isn't plenty, somebody's got to be thrown out of the lifeboat. Somebody's got to be eaten to keep the others alive. . . . Then you can afford ethics, when you have lots of time and somebody else is doing the dirty work.[12]

A recent article in *The Wall Street Journal* is definitive on one aspect of the major medical dilemmas which are facing physicians and, ultimately, every man, woman, and child in our society. After citing a gripping example of patient neglect due to the unavailability of a bed in an intensive care unit in a leading hospital, the article explains that in order to deal with the problem of too many patients and not enough beds in intensive care:

> Doctors are turning to an old battlefield policy: triage. In wartime, doctors and nurses used triage to ration scarce medical care to the wounded. They denied care to those whose wounds could wait or those who were beyond help and concentrated on the neediest who might still be saved.[13]

Today, rather than restricting it to the battlefield, "'Triage is an everyday occurrence in the ICU,' says Daniel Teres, director of the adult critical care division at Baystate Medical Center in Springfield, Massachusetts."[14]

According to the journal, emergency rooms have closed their doors, at times, to those who need immediate and intensive care because there is no room. The quality of care for those who are given beds is sometimes poor because of a shortage in experienced nursing care.

The why of the intensive care dilemma is not hard to assess: too few nurses who are trained on this level and an increase in the elderly; while, "in many urban areas, ICU beds are increasingly occupied by patients with gunshot wounds or acquired immune deficiency syndrome."

The article concludes with a question: "'Are we going to put in [into intensive care units] people with terminal malignancies, AIDS, other irreversible diseases?' asks Bellevue's Dr. Garay. 'That is a societal decision. I don't think doctors should make it alone.'"[15]

The questions are out there: who shall live and who shall die and who shall make the decisions? And if the measure of a society is how it treats the helpless, we have a major test of our morality ahead of us. It is not hard to conceive of a day when decisions will routinely be made which control population growth, cope with a scarcity of medical care, and appeal to just plain monetary greed by killing the young and the old, the sick and the dying, and, eventually, by killing anyone society feels at that time is life unworthy of life.

But God Still Guides

The water is indeed murky. But even when we cannot see, God sees and he will guide our thinking and our actions if we truly want that guidance. For God is not some nice thought or a pleasant concept. He is a Person in whose image we were created. He is real and has supernatural powers. In a day when the reality of Satan's activity in this world is readily acknowledged, it is amazing to me, in just my own counseling practice, how quickly non-Christians acknowledge the power of Satan and how fearful believers are to admit to any supernatural powers from the King of Kings, Jehovah God. Can the counterfeit be more real than the Real? Can Satan be more real than God?

A woman who is not prone to emotional outbursts or fantasies and is a real believer in Jesus Christ told me an amazing story. When she was a child on a farm in the midwest, she was injured in a farming accident and lost her leg. In those first hours after the accident, she lay in a hospital bed in a small country hospital with her mother sitting helplessly by her bed.

As night approached, she started to hemorrhage profusely. The doctor was called, and she overheard him say to her mother: "She won't last the night."

Shortly after that, she felt a comforting hand on her forehead, smoothing her hair back. She heard a voice say reassuringly: "Go to sleep, Pat. When you wake up in the morning you'll be better." Only her mother was in the room, and neither the hand nor the voice were those of her mother.

The child asked her mother at that point to turn back the sheet so that the "angel" could sit there. The mother saw and heard nothing, but she obeyed the child. Then the mother looked into her daughter's face and saw color where there had been a deathly white only a few minutes before.

The child slept. And when she awoke she was better. Not healed, for she still lost her leg. But she lived.

John Noble, who was taken prisoner during World

War II, found God in a Soviet prison camp. During the course of his imprisonment he was put on a starvation diet. His thought then was that he would die soon and go to be with God. Each day he was brought flavored water. For nine days he went down physically, until he was at the edge of death. But he did not die. Then, according to his own story:

> On the tenth day of starvation, I was stronger than on the ninth, and on the eleventh day stronger than on the tenth!
> To feel that I grew stronger, even though I was still denied food of any kind, gave me renewed confidence in the Lord. If it was the Lord's will that I should live, and grow stronger without even any human food for my body, it meant I no longer had to worry about bread or about anything else. It was manifest that the Lord did not intend that I should die at this time. I had asked for death. He had given me life. Nothing could happen to me now, I knew, unless the Lord permitted it.[16]

While my previously mentioned experience, where I stopped breathing right before surgery, is less dramatic than either that of John Noble or the child who lost her leg, it produced some similar feelings in me. At first I felt my life depended on the physicians' skill and motivation; and, of course, in a sense it did. Yet in that operating room, the overwhelming conviction which kept coming to my mind was that *only* God really controlled life and death. The doctors could perform brilliantly; but if God wanted me, he would take me. On the other hand, the doctors could fail miserably; but if God wanted me to live, I would live. In that I rested. Once again we are brought back to unconditional faith in the unconditional love of God.

The reader must form his or her own conclusions about the potential for the supernatural intervention of God himself in our lives, but it is important that we who are Christians do not minimize the power of God. For when our own powers cease and when we do not understand the will of God in some of the complicated issues of medical ethics, we need to know that there is still a God who will lead and undertake for us. With him we do not need to fear making major and permanent mistakes. In ignorance we may turn off a respirator too soon, but he can still keep the person alive. Or we may use a respirator for *too long* a time, but he can still take the person home to himself in spite of us.

Never, of course, is the sovereignty of God to be used as an excuse for sloppiness or for failure to obey the known will of God. It would be wrong, for example, to refuse antibiotics when you have pneumonia just because "God can heal me, so I don't need to go to doctors." It seems consistent with Scripture to accept resources which God makes available to us. Not to do so would be to test God, even as Satan tested Christ when he tempted him to cast himself down and "prove" that he was truly the Son of God. Nor is the sovereignty of God ever to be used as an excuse for failing to seek out the will of God. For example, if we refuse to turn off a respirator when all reasonable medical indicators are to do so, with the attitude that we'll "just leave it all to God" rather than seek his will and make a decision, God may well *not* intervene.

But God who is *sovereign* is also *good* and, when we truly want his sovereign will in our lives, he will come in and undertake in spite of our human frailty and our misguided decisions. All he asks from us is that we give ourselves to him, totally and completely. Then, in the thought of that old hymn by A.B. Simpson, "I take, he undertakes."

If God is so miraculously real in this world, how much more must he be in heaven. Someday, when we go to be with him, we shall find out that all the things we cherished so much on this earth, while important, were only shadows of that heavenly reality. Now we know in part. Now we experience joy only as it filters through our pain. Then we shall know in full; and we shall know unfiltered joy. Heaven will be more real than earth ever was.

In her book *Legacy of a Pack Rat*, Ruth Bell Graham gives us a glimpse of the reality of heaven as viewed through a crack in the spiritual ceiling of earth:

The room was quiet and semidarkened. The elderly lady lying against the pillows listened as her son, Robert [Armistead], talked of the family, her friends, and other things of interest to her.

She looked forward to his daily visits. Madison, where he lived, was not far from Nashville, and Robert spent as much time as he could with his mother, knowing, as ill as she was, each visit might be his last. As he talked, his eyes took in every detail of her loved face, every line—and there were more lines than curves now—the white hair, the tired, still loving eyes. When time came to leave, he kissed her gently on her forehead, assuring her he would be back the next day.

Arriving back at his home in Madison, he found Robin, his seventeen-year-old, was ill with a strange fever. The next few days his time was completely taken up between his son and his mother.

He did not tell his mother of Robin's illness. He was her oldest grandson—the pride and joy of her life.

Then, suddenly, Robin was gone. His death shocked the whole community as well as his family. The whole thing had happened so quickly. And seventeen is too young to die.

As soon as the funeral was over, Mr. Armistead hurried to his mother's bedside, praying nothing in his manner would betray the fact he had just buried his firstborn. It would be more than his mother could take in her condition.

The doctor was in the room as he entered. His mother was lying with her eyes closed.

"She is in a coma," the doctor said gently. He knew something of the strain this man had been under, his faithful visits to his mother, the death of his son, the funeral from which he had just come. . . .

The doctor put his hand on Mr. Armistead's shoulder in wordless sympathy.

"Just sit beside her," he said, "she might come to. . . ."
And he left them together.

Mr. Armistead's heart was heavy as he sat in the gathering twilight.

He lit the lamp on the bedside table, and the shadows receded.

Soon she opened her eyes, and smiled in recognition, she put her hand on her son's knee.

"Bob . . ." she said his name lovingly—and drifted into a coma again.

Quietly Mr. Armistead sat on, his hand over hers, his eyes never leaving her face. After awhile there was a slight movement on the pillow.

His mother's eyes were open and there was a far-off look in them, as if she were seeing beyond the room. A look of wonder passed over her face.

"I see Jesus," she exclaimed, adding, "why there's Father . . . and there's Mother. . . ."

And then,

"And there's Robby! I didn't know Robby had died. . . ."

Her hand patted her son's knee gently.

"Poor Bob . . ." she said softly, and was gone.[17]

"At the Gate of the Year"

As we approach the end of this century we may feel that through our advances in science we are well on our way to solving all of man's problems. Yet, with many of the seeming solutions which we have discovered, we have merely multiplied the problems as a result. Leon Kass writes:

> Thoughtful men have long known that the campaign for the technological conquest of nature, conducted under the banner of modern science, would someday train its guns against the commanding officer, man himself. That day is fast approaching, if not already here.[18]

In our transition into the twenty-first century, many of us cling to modern medicine to cure and at the same time we run from its technological nightmare. And at times, while we know that Jesus Christ is the Light of the world, there seems to be a deep fog preventing us from seeing that Light as clearly and as quickly as we would like, and we become enthralled with easy answers. Then we come back full circle to resting in the sovereignty of a loving God.

As we stand at the gate of a new century, it is awesome to be alive. Not in our wildest imaginations can we with any accuracy conceive of what it will be like at the outset of the twenty-second century. For now, the question marks of the twentieth century are quite enough to cope with.

Sometimes in all of our lives the darkness seems close to engulfing us. Amy Carmichael has a word for such times:

> Once when I was climbing at night in the forest before there was a made path, I learned what the word meant, Psalm 119:105: "Thy word is a *lantern* to my path." I had a lantern and had to hold it very low or I should certainly have slipped on those rough rocks. We don't walk spiritually by electric light but by a hand lantern. And a lantern shows only the next step—not several ahead.[19]

There are times in life when the darkness seems complete, when we feel that, with all of our best efforts, we just don't have the answers we need to deal with our questions or the solutions we crave to solve our problems. We feel that, through no fault of our own, we walk in the darkness; and that Light, which we know is out there somewhere, seems totally obscured by a dark fog.

As the Nazis moved in power across Europe, on Christmas day, 1939, King George VI broadcasted his annual message to the English people who at that point were beginning to feel completely surrounded by the darkness of Nazism. In his speech the king quoted the following lines from Minnie Louise Haskins:

> I said to the man who stood at the gate of the year, "Give me a light that I may tread safely into the unknown." And he replied, "Go out into the darkness and put your hand into the hand of God. That shall be to you better than light and safer than a known way!"[20]

Notes

Acknowledgments

1. Amy Carmichael, *Kohila* (Fort Washington, Penn.: Christian Literature Crusade, n.d.), 112.
2. Richard E. Day, *The Shadow of the Broad Brim* (Valley Forge, Penn.: Judson Press, 1934), 198.
3. Winston Churchill, *The Second World War*, vol. 1, *The Gathering Storm* (Boston: Houghton Mifflin Co., 1976), 201.

Preface

1. Amy Carmichael, *Gold Cord* (Fort Washington, Penn.: Christian Literature Crusade, 1947), 28. (©1932 Dohnavur Fellowship; used by permission.)
2. Ibid., 31.
3. Martin Niemöller, as quoted in Dr. Franklin H. Lihell, "Lest We Forget: The Need to Expose Holocaust Myths, Plain Fiction and Lies," *The Jewish Times* (May 1, 1986).

Chapter 1: "... And I Was Being So Good"

1. Claude Lévy and Paul Tillard, quoted in Philip Hallie, *Lest Innocent Blood Be Shed* (New York: Harper Colophon Books, 1980), 275.
2. Derrick Sington, quoted in Walter Laqueur, *The Terrible*

Secret Suppression of the Truth About Hitler's "Final Solution" (Boston: Little, Brown and Co., 1980), 1.

3. Ibid.

4. Robert Proctor, *Racial Hygiene, Medicine Under the Nazis* (Cambridge, Mass.: Harvard University Press, 1988), 184.

5. Ibid.

6. Ibid., 185.

7. Ibid.

8. Ibid., 180.

9. Jane Gross, "What Medical Care the Poor Can Have: Lists Are Drawn Up," *New York Times* (March 27, 1989), 1.

10. Ibid.

11. John Elson, "Rationing Medical Care," *Time* (May 15, 1989), 86.

12. Ibid, 84.

13. Allan Parachini, "79 Doctors in California Survey Admit to Euthanasia," *Los Angeles Times* (February 25, 1988), sec. V, 1.

14. Sidney H. Wanzer, et. al., "The Physician's Responsibility Toward Hopelessly Ill Patients," *The New England Journal of Medicine*, vol. 320 (March 30, 1989), 844.

15. William Byron Forbush, ed., *Fox's Book of Martyrs* (Philadelphia: Universal Book and Bible House, 1926), 6.

16. Ibid., 11.

17. Ibid.

18. C. S. Lewis, *The Problem of Pain* (New York: Macmillan Co., 1952), 105.

19. Amy Carmichael, *Rose From Brier* (Ft. Washington, Penn.: Christian Literature Crusade, 1972), xii. (©1933 Dohnavur Fellowship; used by permission.)

20. G. Campbell Morgan, *The Analyzed Bible, The Book of Job* (New York: Fleming H. Revell Co., 1909), 84.

21. Annette E. Dumbach and Jud Newborn, *Shattering the German Night, The Story of the White Rose* (Boston: Little, Brown and Co., 1986), 90.

Chapter 2: A Decision to Love

1. Philip Hallie, *Lest Innocent Blood Be Shed* (New York: Harper Colophon Books, 1980), 18.

2. Ibid., 20.

3. Ibid., 120.

4. Albert Speer, *Inside the Third Reich, Memoirs* , trans. Richard

and Clara Winston (New York: Macmillan, Collier, 1970), 523-24.

5. Alan Redpath, *The Royal Route to Heaven, Studies in First Corinthians* (Old Tappan, N.J.: Fleming H. Revell Co., 1960), 156-57.

6. Anthony Cave Brown, *Bodyguard of Lies* (New York: Harper and Row, Bantam, 1976), 798.

7. A. R. Fausset, *A Commentary (Critical, Experimental and Practical) on the Old and New Testaments, 1 Corinthians—Revelation* (Grand Rapids, Mich.: Wm. B. Eerdmans, 1945), 591.

8. Amy Carmichael, *If* (Fort Washington, Penn.: Christian Literature Crusade; London, SPCK, n.d.), 44. (©1938 Dohnavur Fellowship; used by permission.)

9. Adam Clarke, *A Commentary and Critical Notes, The Old and New Testaments*, vol. 3 (New York: Abingdon-Cokesbury Press, n.d.), 167.

10. Ed Larson and Beth Spring, "Life-defying Acts," *Christianity Today* (February 20, 1987), 53.

11. Ibid.

12. Peter Singer and Deane Wells, *Making Babies, The New Science and Ethics of Conception* (New York: Charles Scribner's Sons, 1985), 176.

13. William Shakespeare, "Sonnet 94," in C. J. Hill, ed., *The Complete Plays and Poems of William Shakespeare* (Cambridge, Mass.: Houghton Mifflin Co., 1942), 1386.

Chapter 3: Arsenal of Words

1. Leon Howard, Louis B. Wright, Carl Bode, *American Heritage, An Anthology and Interpretive Survey of Our Literature*, vol. 1 (Boston: D. C. Heath and Co., 1955), 240.

2. Ibid., 247.

3. Viktor E. Frankl, M.D., *The Doctor and the Soul* (New York: Random House, Vintage, 1973), xxi.

4. William L. Shirer, *The Rise and Fall of the Third Reich* (New York: Simon and Schuster, 1959), 100.

5. Ibid.

6. Stewart Spencer and Barry Millington, "Selected Letters of Richard Wagner," *The New Yorker* (October 1988), 108.

7. Shirer, *Rise and Fall*, 101.

8. Ibid., 236.

9. Martin Luther, "On Mistreating Jews," in Ewald M. Plass, ed., *Luther Says, Anthology*, vol. 2 (St. Louis, Mo.: Concordia

Publishing House, 1959), 683.

10. Martin Luther, "The Bad Effects of Persecution," in Ibid., 2120.

11. Ewald M. Plass, ed. *Luther Says, Anthology*, vol. 3 (St. Louis, Mo.: Concordia Publishing House, 1959), 1621.

12. Roland H. Bainton, *Here I Stand, A Life of Martin Luther* (New York: New American Library, 1977), 297-98.

13. Annette E. Dumbach and Jud Newborn, *Shattering the German Night,The Story of the White Rose* (Boston: Little Brown and Co., 1986), 108-09.

14. Warren T. Reich, ed. *Encyclopedia of Bioethics*, vol. 1 (New York: Macmillan, Free Press, 1978), 830.

15. Ibid., 835.

16. Ibid.

17. Robert Lifton, *The Nazi Doctors, Medical Killing and the Psychology of Genocide* (New York: Basic Books, 1986), 22.

18. Ibid., 23.

19. Ibid., 65.

20. Ibid., 46.

21. Ibid., 47.

22. Christopher Nolan, *Under the Eye of the Clock* (New York: St. Martin's Press, 1987), 119.

23. Ibid., 148.

24. Ibid., 53.

25. Ibid., 82.

26. Ibid., 84.

27. Raymond S. Duff, M.D., and A. G. M. Campbell, M.D. "Moral and Ethical Dilemmas in the Special-Care Nursery," *The New England Journal of Medicine*, vol. 289 (October 15, 1973), 890.

Chapter 4: Enabling Evil

1. Ann Tusa and John Tusa, *The Nuremberg Trial* (New York: Macmillan, Atheneum, 1983), 236-37.

2. Robert Lifton, *The Nazi Doctors, Medical Killing and the Psychology of Genocide* (New York: Basic Books, 1986), 418.

3. Gerald Astor, *The Last Nazi, The Life and Times of Dr. Joseph Mengele* (New York: Donald I. Fine, 1985), 84.

4. Robert Proctor, *Racial Hygiene, Medicine Under the Nazis* (Cambridge, Mass.: Harvard University Press, 1988), 240-241.

5. Ibid.

6. Lifton, *Nazi Doctors*, 430.

Chapter 5: "If I Should Die Before I Wake . . ."

1. Hardin Craig, ed., *Jonathan Swift Selections* (New York: Charles Scribner's Sons, 1924), 370.

2. Ibid., 368-69.

3. James K. Hoffmeier, ed., *Abortion, A Christian Understanding and Response* (Grand Rapids, Mich.: Baker Book House, 1987), 53.

4. Ibid., 50., see author's note 2.

5. Ibid., 52.

6. Ibid., 59.

7. C. H. Spurgeon, *The Treasury of David*, vol. 3b (Grand Rapids, Mich.: Zondervan Publishing House, 1976), 280-81.

8. David M'Laren, quoted in Ibid.

9. J. A. Thompson, *The Book of Jeremiah* (Grand Rapids, Mich.: Wm. B. Eerdmans, 1980), 145.

10. John Bright, "Jeremiah's Call and Commission," *The Anchor Bible*, vol. 3 (New York: Doubleday and Co., 1978), 3.

11. Andrew W. Blackwood, Jr., *Commentary on Jeremiah* (Waco, Texas: Word Books, 1980), 37.

12. Ibid., 37.

13. C. F. Keil and F. Delitzsch, *Commentary on the Old Testament, The Pentateuch*, vol. 2 (Grand Rapids, Mich.: Wm. B. Eerdmans, 1981), 134-35.

14. Adam Clarke, *A Commentary and Critical Notes, The Holy Bible* vol. 1 (New York: Abingdon-Cokesbury Press, n.d.), 412.

15. S. Rickly Christian, *The Woodland Hills Tragedy* (Westchester, Ill.: Crossway Books, 1985), 137.

16. Donald S. Smith, comp., *The Silent Scream*, ed. Don Tanner (Anaheim, Calif.: American Portrait Films Books, 1985), 16.

17. Leon R. Kass, M.D., *Toward a More Natural Science: Biology and Human Affairs* (New York: Macmillan, Free Press, 1985), 229.

18. Hoffmeier, *Abortion*, 201.

19. Christian, *Woodland Hills Tragedy*, 61.

20. Ibid.

21. Don Feder, "Sick of Death," *Pentecostal Evangel* (November 27, 1988), 12.

22. Ibid.

23. Hoffmeier, *Abortion*, 168-69.

24. Francis Schaeffer and C. Everett Koop, M.D., *Whatever Happened to the Human Race?* (Old Tappan, N.J.: Fleming H. Revell Co., 1979), 37.

25. Ann Tusa and John Tusa, *The Nuremberg Trial* (New York: Macmillan, Atheneum, 1984), 87.

Chapter 6: Opening Pandora's Box

1. Howard L. Goodkind, et. al., eds., *The Young Children's Encyclopedia*, vol. 12 (Chicago: Encyclopaedia Britannica,1977), 12.

2. Francis Schaeffer and C. Everett Koop, M.D., *Whatever Happened to the Human Race?* (Old Tappan, N.J.: Fleming H. Revell, 1979), 36.

3. Richard John Neuhaus, "The Return of Eugenics," American Jewish Committee, 1988, *Commentary*, vol. 85 (April 1988), 24-25.

4. Kathleen McAuliffe, "A Startling Fount of Healing," *U.S. News* (Nov 3, 1986), 68-70. See also John D. Arras and Shlomo Shinnar, "Anencephalic Newborns as Organ Donors: A Critique," *Journal of the American Medical Association* (April 15, 1988), 2284-85.

5. Richard N. Ostling, "Technology and the Womb," *Time* (March 23, 1987), 59.

6. Leon R. Kass, M.D., *Toward a More Natural Science: Biology and Human Affairs* (New York: Macmillan, Free Press, 1985), 47-48.

7. Ibid., 72.

8. Christine Gorman, "A Balancing Act of Life and Death," *Time* (February 1, 1988), 49. See also, Kim A. Lawton, "Fetal-tissue Transplants Stir Controversy," *Christianity Today* (March 18, 1988), 52.

9. Ibid. See also Joe Levine, "Help from the Unborn," *Time* (January 12, 1987), 62.

10. James Manney and John C. Blattner, *Death in the Nursery: Secret Crime of Infanticide* (Ann Arbor, Mich.: Servant Books, 1984), 117.

11. Ibid., 118.

12. Joseph Fletcher, quoted in Melinda Delahoyde, *Fighting for Life, Defending the Newborn's Right to Live* (Ann Arbor, Mich.: Servant Books, 1984), 11.

13. Joseph Fletcher, quoted in D. Alan Shewmon, M.D., "Active Voluntary Euthanasia: A Needless Pandora's Box," *Issues in Law and Medicine*, vol. 3, 1987, 231.

14. C. Everett Koop, quoted in Ibid., 239.

15. Robert Lifton, *The Nazi Doctors, Medical Killing and the Psychology of Genocide* (New York: Basic Books, 1986),15-16.

16. Leo Alexander, M.D., "Medical Science Under Dictatorship" *New England Journal of Medicine*, vol. 241 (July 14, 1949), 45.

Chapter 7: Touching the Face of Evil

1. Gerald J. Gruman, "Death and Dying: Euthanasia and Sustaining Life," *Encyclopedia of Bioethics:* vol. 1, ed. Warren T. Reich (NewYork: Macmillan, 1978), 261-62.

2. Ibid., 262.

3. Ibid., 269.

4. Adolf Meyer, *The Commonsense Psychiatry of Dr. Adolf Meyer* (New York: McGraw Hill Book Co., 1948), 83.

5. Berlin Correspondent, "Problems of Heredity," *Journal of the American Medical Association,* vol. 105 (July 29,1935), 1051.

6. Ibid.

7. Paul Popenoe, "The Progress of Eugenic Sterilization," *The Journal of Heredity,* vol. 25 (January 1934), 24.

8. Ibid., 25-26.

9. Kenneth Asp, Independent Researcher, Interview (February 18, 1989).

10. Fredric Wertham, M.D., *A Sign for Cain, An Exploration of Human Violence* (New York: Macmillan, 1966), 153.

11. Ibid., 157.

12. Ibid., 159.

13. Berlin Correspondent, "The Right of Putting Incurable Patients Out of the Way," *Journal of the American Medical Association,* vol. 75 (October 2, 1920), 1283.

14. Leo Alexander, M.D., "Medical Science Under Dictatorship," *New England Journal of Medicine,* vol. 241 (July 14, 1949), 39.

15. D. Alan Shewmon, "Active Voluntary Euthanasia: A Needless Pandora's Box," *Issues in Law and Medicine,* vol. 3 (1987), 228. See also, F. Wertham, *A Sign for Cain,* 162.

16. Alexander, "Medical Science Under Dictatorship," 39.

17. Wertham, *A Sign for Cain,* 187.

18. Ibid., 165.

19. Christoph Hupeland, quoted in Ibid., 153.

20. Shewmon, "Active Voluntary Euthanasia," 228.

21. Foster Kennedy, M.D., "The Problem of Social Control of the Congenital Defective," *The American Journal of Psychiatry,* vol. 99 (July 1942), 14.

22. Ibid.

23. Quoted in Richard Neuhaus, "The Return of Eugenics," *Commentary,* vol. 85 (April 1988), 20.

24. J. K. M. Gevers, "Legal Developments Concerning Active Euthanasia on Request in the Netherlands" *Bioethics ,* vol. 1, no. 2 (1987), 161.

25. H. J. de Roy van Zuydewijn, Secretary to the Health Council, "Euthanasia in the Netherlands," The Hague (March 23, 1987), 2.

26. Dr. Pieter V. Admiraal, address at the fiftieth anniversary celebration of the Voluntary Euthanasia Society, Holland (April 14, 1985).

27. Jeane Tromp Meesters, "The Member's Aid Service of the Dutch Association for Voluntary Euthanasia," *The Euthanasia Review*, vol. 1 (3) Fall 1986, Human Sciences Press.

28. "Euthanasia Across the North Sea," (available from the Consulate General of the Netherlands, New York, Los Angeles).

29. "Aide mémoire regarding euthanasia in the Netherlands," 2 (available from the Consulate General of the Netherlands, New York, Los Angeles).

30. Shewmon, "Active Voluntary Euthanasia," 229. See also A. Parachini, "The Netherlands Debates the Legal Limits of Euthanasia," *Los Angeles Times* (July 5, 1987), sec. VI, 1.

31. M. E. Conolly, M.D., "The Death of Man, The Case Against Euthanasia," unpublished manuscript, June 13, 1988, 5.

32. Richard Fenigsen, "A Case Against Dutch Euthanasia," *The Hastings Center Report*, vol. 19, no. 1 (January/February 1989), 24.

33. Ibid.

34. Ibid., 26.

35. Alexander, "Medical Science Under Dictatorship," 45. See also Gaylin, et. al, "Doctors Must Not Kill," *Journal of the American Medical Association*, vol. 259 (April 8, 1988), 2139-40.

36. Ibid., 44.

37. Leon R. Kass, M.D., *Toward a More Natural Science: Biology and Human Affairs* (New York: Macmillan, Free Press, 1985), 89.

38. Abraham Lincoln, quoted in Ibid., 90.

39. Anthony Cave Brown, *Bodyguard of Lies* (New York: Harper and Row, Bantam, 1976), 389.

40. Philip Hallie, *Lest Innocent Blood Be Shed* (New York: Harper Colophon Books, 1980), 126.

41. Leo Alexander, M.D., "Temporal Laws and Medical Ethics in Conflict," *New England Journal of Medicine*, vol. 289 (August 9, 1973), 324.

42. C. S. Lewis, *The Problem of Pain* (New York: Macmillan, 1952), 105.

43. C. S. Lewis, *A Grief Observed* (New York: Seabury Press, 1963), 36.

Chapter 8: In His Time

1. Matthew F. Conolly, M.D., "Do Not Go Gentle Into That Good Night: The Case Against Euthanasia," *Los Angeles Herald Examiner* (December 19, 1982), sec. F, 1.

2. Arthur Pink, *Gleanings in Genesis* (Chicago: Moody Press, 1922), 115.

3. Andrew Fuller, quoted in Ibid.

4. Billy Graham, *Facing Death and the Life After* (Dallas: Word, 1987), 134.

5. Wanzer, et al., "The Physician's Responsibility Toward Hopelessly Ill Patients," *The New England Journal of Medicine* (March 30, 1989), 848.

6. W. Graham Scroggie, *The Psalms* (London: Pickering and Inglis Ltd., 1951), vol. 4, 45.

7. Ibid., 46.

8. Ibid.

9. Rabbi Yitzchok Adlerstein, Director of Jewish Studies at Yeshiva University of Los Angeles, Interview (March 14, 1989).

10. Annette E. Dumbach and Jud Newborn, *Shattering the German Night, The Story of the White Rose* (Boston: Little, Brown and Co., 1986), 203.

11. Richard G. Benton, *Death and Dying, Principles and Practices in Patient Care* (New York: Van Nortrand Reinhold Co., 1978), 18-19.

12. Ibid.

13. Graham, *Facing Death*, 145-47.

14. Benton, *Death and Dying*, 6.

15. Ibid., 7.

16. Ibid.

17. Joseph Bayly, "A Psalm on Viewing the River," *Psalms of My Life* (Elgin, Ill.: David C. Cook Publishing Co., 1987), 36. Used by permission of David C. Cook Pub. Co.

18. Thomas A. Shannon and JoAnn Manfra, ed. *Law and Bioethics, Texts with Commentary on Major U.S. Court Decisions* (New York: Paulist Press, 1982), 165.

19. Ibid., 155.

20. John White, "A Concluding Thought," *Decision* (May 1989), 35.

21. Benton, *Death and Dying*, 11.

22. Ibid.

23. Leo Alexander, M.D. "Temporal Laws and Medical Ethics

in Conflict," *The New England Journal of Medicine*, vol. 289 (August 9, 1973), 325.

24. Ann Tusa and John Tusa, *The Nuremberg Trial* (New York: Atheneum, 1984), 198.

25. Ibid., 473.

Chapter 9: Question Marks

1. Alfred J. Crick, exposition on the Book of John, from author's personally taped sermon.

2. David S. Wyman, *The Abandonment of the Jews: America and the Holocaust, 1941-1945* (New York: Pantheon Books, 1984), 40-41.

3. Elie Wiesel, *Night*, trans. Stella Rodway (New York: Bantam Books, 1960), 4.

4. Ibid., 8.

5. Joy Horowitz, "Dr. Amnio, UCLA's Controversial New Chief of Obstetrics, Takes Risks Others Won't, Saves Babies Others Can't," *Los Angeles Times Magazine* (April 23, 1989), 12.

6. Hubert Humphrey, as quoted by KCET (Los Angeles, Calif.) television program *Ethics in America*, "Do Unto Others" recorded by author, February 13, 1988.

7. Frederick E. Werbelland and Thurston Clarke, *Lost Hero: The Mystery of Raoul Wallenberg* (New York: McGraw-Hill Book Co., 1982), 192.

8. Kati Marton, *Wallenberg* (New York: Random House, 1982), 96.

9. John Bierman, *Righteous Gentile, The Story of Raoul Wallenberg, Missing Hero of the Holocaust* (New York: The Viking Press, 1981), 83.

10. Annette E. Dumbach and Jud Newborn, *Shattering the German Night, The Story of the White Rose* (Boston: Little, Brown and Co., 1986), 88.

11. Dietrich Bonhoeffer, *Letters and Papers from Prison*, ed. Eberhard Bethge (New York: Collier Books, Macmillan, 1971), 14.

12. Ian Jones, M.D., head of obstetrics and gynecology, Scripps Clinic, La Jolla, Calif., Interview, January 9, 1989.

13. Alan L. Otten, "Intensive Care Units Are Neglecting Patients Because of Crowding," *The Wall Street Journal*, Western edition (May 23, 1989), 1.

14. Ibid.

15. Ibid.

16. John Noble and Glenn D. Everett, *I Found God in Soviet*

Russia (Grand Rapids, Mich.: Zondervan Publishing House, 1959), 44-45.

17. Ruth Bell Graham, *Legacy of a Pack Rat* (Nashville: Thomas Nelson Publishers, Oliver Nelson, 1989), 218-20.

18. Kass, *More Natural Science*, 43.

19. Amy Carmichael, *Candles in the Dark* (Ft. Washington, Penn.: Christian Literature Crusade; London, SPCK, 1981), 43. (©1981 Dohnavur Fellowship; used by permission.)

20. Minnie Louise Haskins, *God Knows*. Quoted by King George VI in a Christmas broadcast, 25 December, 1939, *The Oxford Dictionary of Quotations* (Oxford Press, 1953).

Suggested Reading

Anger, Per. *With Raoul Wallenberg in Budapest.* New York: Holocaust Pubns., 1981. Ambassador Per Anger's story of Raoul Wallenberg in Budapest from the point of view of a fellow diplomat who was there with him.

Astor, Gerald. *The "Last" Nazi: The Life and Times of Dr. Joseph Mengele.* New York: D. I. Fine, 1985. An insightful biography of that most notorious of Nazi doctors.

Bayly, Joseph. *The Last Thing We Talk About* (Former title: *A View From a Hearse*). Elgin, Ill.: Cook, 1973. Helpful book on dealing with the death of a loved one.

Benton, Richard G. *Death and Dying.* New York: Van Nostrand Reinhold, 1978. Factual, informative book on dying and related topics—good reference material.

Bierman, John. *Righteous Gentile: The Story of Raoul Wallenberg, Missing Hero of the Holocaust.* New York: Viking, 1981. Balanced account of the hero of Budapest during World War II.

Blattner, John C. and James Manney. *Death in the Nursery: The Secret Crime of Infanticide.* Ann Arbor, Mich.: Servant Pubns., 1984. Excellent and balanced presentation of the treatment of the newborn as it relates to infanticide. Good reading for parents who face serious illness in a newborn.

Bonhoeffer, Dietrich. *Letters and Papers from Prison.* New York: Macmillan, Collier, 1971. The thought of a famous Lutheran pastor who was imprisoned and executed for his resistance to the growth of Nazism in his country, Germany. Inspirational.

Brinkley, David. *Washington Goes to War.* New York: Knopf, 1988. Vivid portrayal of Washington D.C. during World War II.

Brown, Anthony Cave. *Bodyguard of Lies.* New York: Bantam Bks., 1975. Espionage during World War II portrayed in an interesting and informative style.

Califano, Joseph A., Jr. *America's Health Care Revolution: Who Lives? Who Dies? Who Pays?* New York: Random Hse., 1986. Former Secretary of Health, Education and Welfare writes about the revolution in health services that the United States is undergoing.

Carmichael, Amy. *Candle in the Dark.* Ft. Washington, Penn.: Christian Lit. Crusade, 1981. Inspirational essay.

Christian, S. Rickly. *Woodland Hills Tragedy.* Westchester, Ill.: Crossway Bks., 1985. The story of the finding of 16,433 fetuses in a container in Woodland Hills, California, and an analysis of the implications of such a find.

Cousins, Norman. *Anatomy of an Illness: As Perceived by the Patient.* New York: Norton, 1979. A personal experience of recovery from illness.

Delahoyde, Melinda. *Fighting for Life: Defending the Newborn's Right to Live.* Ann Arbor, Mich.: Servant Pbns., 1984. Overall picture of infanticide as it relates to our view of the care of the newborn.

Dumbach, Annette E. and Jud Newborn. *Shattering the German Night: The Story of the White Rose.* Boston: Little, Brown and Co., 1986. Moving and inspiring story of the courage of students in Munich who resisted the Nazis and gave their lives for the Resistance.

Fabrizius, Peter, Max Knight, and Joseph Fabry. *One and One Make Three.* Berkeley: Benmir Bks., 1988. Fascinating story of two young men who escaped from Austria after Hitler's invasion. Excellent reading.

Frank, Anne. *The Diary of a Young Girl*. New York: Doubleday and Co., 1967. The diary of a young Jewish girl who was hidden from the Nazis, but who was later imprisoned in Bergen-Belsen concentration camp where she died. A wonderful and even positive book. Every teenager should read it.

Frankl, Viktor E. *The Doctor and the Soul: From Psychotherapy to Logotherapy*. New York: Random Hse, Vintage Bks., 1973. A moving story of a Jewish doctor's experiences in Hitler's camps along with a brief description of logotherapy—a therapy of meaning.

Gies, Miep with Alison L. Gold. *Anne Frank Remembered: The Story of the Woman Who Helped to Hide the Frank Family*. New York: Simon and Schuster, 1987. A hauntingly beautiful story of compassion against the backdrop of the hatred of the Holocaust. Also informative relating to the Resistance in Holland.

Graham, Billy. *Facing Death and the Life After*. Waco, Tex.: Word Bks., 1987. Offers biblical truths relating to death and heaven—a practical and inspirational look at difficult subjects.

Graham, Ruth Bell. *Legacy of a Pack Rat*. Nashville: Nelson, 1989. A montage of poetry, prayer, and quotes—collected by the wife of evangelist Billy Graham—relating to this high-tech age.

Hallie, Philip. *Lest Innocent Blood Be Shed*. New York: Harper and Row, Colophon, 1979. The remarkable story of Le Chambon, a small village in France which resisted the Nazis in a dramatic way.

Hoffmeier, James K., ed. *Abortion, A Christian Understanding and Response*. Grand Rapids, Mich.: Baker Bk Hse., 1987. Essays on abortion and related topics, written from a scholarly point of view.

Kass, Leon R. *Toward a More Natural Science: Biology and Human Affairs*. New York: Macmillan, Free Press, 1985. Scholarly analysis on humanness in an age of high-tech medicine.

Koop, C. Everett. *The Right to Live; The Right to Die.* Wheaton, Ill.: Tyndale, 1976. Issues relating to the sanctity of life. Well thought out and presented.

Laqueur, Walter. *The Terrible Secret.* Boston: Little, Brown and Co., 1980. Comprehensive but readable work on genocide and the world's reaction to it during World War II.

Levi, Primo. *If This Is a Man: Remembering Auschwitz.* New York: Simon and Schuster, Summit Bks., 1985. Personal narrative of his ten months spent in a Nazi death camp and the confusion he experienced following liberation.

Lewis, C. S. *A Grief Observed.* New York: Harper and Row, Seabury Press, 1961. His views on death—particularly the death of his wife.

———. *The Problem of Pain.* New York: Macmillan, 1962. Scholarly discussion of pain from a Christian point of view.

Lifton, Robert Jay. *The Nazi Doctors: Medical Killing and the Psychology of Genocide.* New York: Harper and Row, Basic Bks., 1986. A must for anyone who wants to understand the "why" of the Holocaust.

Manchester, William. *The Last Lion; Winston Spencer Churchill: Alone 1932-1940.* Boston: Little, Brown and Co., 1988. The biographical volume covering the period of history preceding the entry of the United States into World War II.

Marton, Kati. *Wallenberg.* New York: Random Hse., 1982. Warmly written biography of Raoul Wallenberg.

Mitscherlich, Alexander and Fred Mielke. *The Death Doctors.* London: Elek Bks., 1962. Data relating to the medical experiments of the Nazi doctors.

———. *Doctors of Infamy: The Story of the Nazi Medical Crimes.* New York: Henry Schuman, 1949. Good overall picture of the medical experimentation and the medicalized killing ordered by the Third Reich.

Mosher, Steven W. *Broken Earth: The Rural Chinese.* New York: Macmillan, Free Press, 1983. Controversial account of rural life in China, including attitudes regarding fetal life.

Muller-Hill, Benno, *Murderous Science: Elimination by Scientific Selection of Jews, Gypsies, and Others, Germany 1933-45.* trans. George R. Fraser. New York: Oxford Univ. Press, 1988.

Nolan, Christopher. *Under the Eye of the Clock.* New York: Macmillan, St. Martin's Press, 1987. A story of triumph over physical disabilities.

Pifer, Alan and Lydia Bronte. *Our Aging Society.* New York: Norton, 1986. A look at aging in this decade.

Powell, John. *Abortion: The Silent Holocaust.* Allen, Tex.: Tabor Pub., Argus Comm., 1981. A strong pro-life approach. Very readable.

Proctor, Robert N. *Medicine Under the Nazis.* Cambridge, Mass.: Harvard Univ. Press, 1988. Story of how Nazi scientists contributed to the Holocaust. Factual and incisive. Also incorporates the views of Nazi scientists with those in other parts of the world.

Reich, Warren T., ed. *Encyclopedia of Bioethics.* 4 vols. Macmillan, Free Press, 1978. The "bible" of bioethics and an essential tool for any serious study.

Ryrie, Charles. *A Look at Life After Death.* Chicago: Moody Press, 1977. On life after death as relayed by those who claim to have died and then returned—conservative viewpoint.

Schaeffer, Francis A. and C. Everett Koop. *Whatever Happened to the Human Race.* Old Tappan, N.J.: Fleming H. Revell, 1979. A discussion of human rights as they relate to medical ethics.

Schemmer, Kenneth E., with Dave and Zeta Jackson. *Between Life and Death: The Life Support Dilemma.* Wheaton, Ill.: Victor Bks., 1988. Deals with dying, particularly with regard to life supports, from one Christian doctor's point of view. Thought provoking and informative.

Schlamm, J. Vera. *Pursued*. Ventura, Calif.: Regal Bks., 1986. A personal account from a survivor of the Holocaust who also became a Christian.

Shannon, Thomas A. and JoAnn Manfra, ed. *Law and Bioethics*. Mahwah, New Jersey: Paulist Press, 1984. The text of and discussion on certain major U.S. court decisions which relate to bioethics.

Shirer, William T. *Berlin Diary*. New York: Knopf, 1941. A view of the growth of Nazi Germany as seen from Berlin by one of this century's greatest journalists.

————. *The Nightmare Years, 1930-1940*. Boston: Little, Brown and Co. 1984. A well-known journalist portrays in a first-hand account the build up in Europe during these crucial years.

————. *The Rise and Fall of the Third Reich: A History of Nazi Germany*. New York: Simon and Schuster, Touchstone Bks., 1960. The classic book on the history of Nazi Germany.

————. *Twentieth Century Journey: The Start: 1904-1930*. Boston: Little, Brown and Co., 1976. An autobiographical account of his early years.

Singer, Peter and Jeane Wells. *Making Babies: The New Science and Ethics of Conception*. New York: Scribner, 1985. A summation of current technologies in infertility and related ethical issues. Viewed from a scientific and secular point of view. Readable.

Skoglund, Elizabeth. *A Divine Blessing: A Well Kept Secret of Life's Second Half*. Minneapolis, Minn.: World Wide Pub., 1988. A biblical and inspirational approach to aging.

————. *More than Coping*. Minneapolis, Minn.: World Wide Pub., 1987. Spiritual resources for coping with life's challenge toward change (taken from the lives of C. S. Lewis, Charles Spurgeon, Amy Carmichael and J. Hudson Taylor).

————. *Safety Zones*. Waco, Tx.: Word Books, 1986. The use of persons, places, ideas, and things in order to buffer and refurbish in the middle of the stress and change of our times.

Smith, Donald S., comp., and Don Tanner, ed. *The Silent Scream*. Anaheim, Calif.: American Portrait Films Books, 1985. Text of the film of an actual abortion.

Tournier, Paul. *Creative Suffering*. New York: Harper and Row, 1983. Positive approach to suffering written from a Christian perspective.

Tusa, Ann and John Tusa. *The Nuremberg Trial*. New York: Macmillan, Atheneum, 1984. Factual account of the trial of Nazi war criminals after World War II. Readable—also of interest is its contribution to international law.

Werbell, Frederick E. and Thurston Clarke. *Last Hero*. New York: McGraw Hill, 1982. Biography of Raoul Wallenberg, including an account of his imprisonment in the Soviet Union.

Wertham, Fredric. *A Sign for Cain*. New York: Macmillan, Collier, 1966. Study on violence, with particular sections on the Third Reich.

Wiesel, Elie. *Night*. New York: Bantam Bks., 1960. Provocative personal narrative which should be followed up with further reading by the same author.

Wiesenthal, Simon. *The Murderers Among Us: The Simon Wiesenthal Memoirs*. New York: McGraw Hill, 1967. Story of the famous Nazi hunter, Simon Wiesenthal: his experiences in a concentration camp and his work thereafter. Has been made into an excellent movie.

Wymen, David S. *The Abandonment of the Jews: America and the Holocaust 1941-1945*. New York: Pantheon Bks., 1984. A provocative discussion of the response and lack of response of the United States and Great Britain to the Holocaust.